H.O.P.E. for the Alzheimer's Journey

H.O.P.E.

for the Alzheimer's Journey

*Help, Organization, Preparation,
and Education for the Road Ahead*

CAROL B. AMOS

The Holy Bible, King James Version

Michael G. Boyd and Ronald D. Boyd emails

NEW YORK

LONDON • NASHVILLE • MELBOURNE • VANCOUVER

H.O.P.E. for the Alzheimer's Journey
Help, Organization, Preparation, and Education for the Road Ahead

Published in New York, New York, by Morgan James Publishing. Morgan James is a trademark of Morgan James, LLC. www.MorganJamesPublishing.com

The Morgan James Speakers Group can bring authors to your live event. For more information or to book an event visit The Morgan James Speakers Group at www.TheMorganJamesSpeakersGroup.com.

ISBN 9781683509035 paperback
ISBN 9781683509042 eBook
Library of Congress Control Number: 2017918890

Cover Design by:
Christopher Kirk
www.GFSstudio.com

Interior Design by:
Chris Treccani
www.3dogcreative.net

Author Photo by:
Theresa Knox Photography

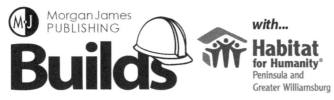

In an effort to support local communities, raise awareness and funds, Morgan James Publishing donates a percentage of all book sales for the life of each book to Habitat for Humanity Peninsula and Greater Williamsburg.

Get involved today! Visit
www.MorganJamesBuilds.com

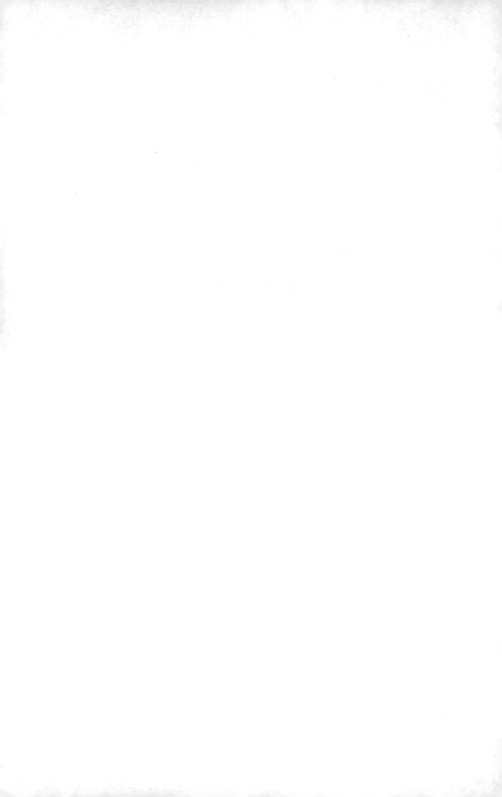

To my parents, Elizabeth and Clarence Boyd

CONTENTS

INTRODUCTION

Honor thy father and thy mother: that thy days may be long upon
the land which the Lord thy God giveth thee
(Exodus 20:12).

My brothers and I were devastated when our mother began displaying signs of Alzheimer's disease, also referred to as Alzheimer's. We became part of the estimated ten million unpaid family members caring for a person with Alzheimer's in the United States[1]. We banded together to face this challenge head-on. I learned about this disease through reading, attending workshops, observing caregivers, and on-the-job training. I have learned from my successes and my failures during this eleven-year period. As a result, I have shared my learning, experience, and encouragement with friends, family, and colleagues as they embarked on their journey. The information has helped them tremendously, and I have learned from their experiences.

H.O.P.E. for the Alzheimer's Journey was written from one caregiver to another to provide help, organization, preparation, and education. Information is shared in an easy-to-read format. The book is a combination of structured information, insights, and personal narratives to demonstrate The Caregiving Principle™. This simple and original framework is introduced to give a deeper understanding of the person with Alzheimer's and the caregiver's role. Many of the ideas and suggestions can be used for caregivers of persons with other health challenges.

Dementia is a group of symptoms characterized by difficulties with cognitive skills that impact the ability of a person to perform everyday activities. Common causes of dementia are:

- Alzheimer's disease
- Vascular dementia
- Dementia with Lewy bodies (DLB)
- Fronto-temporal lobar degeneration (FTLD)
- Parkinson's disease
- Creutzfeldt-Jakob disease
- Mixed dementia—a combination of multiple causes of dementia. Alzheimer's disease and vascular are the most common mixed dementia.

Alzheimer's disease is the most common form of dementia. It accounts for 60 to 80 percent of all dementia cases[2]. Although each person with the disease is unique, and his or her experiences can be different, there are generic symptoms and similarities. This book will focus on the person with Alzheimer's disease. It is an attempt to provoke thought and offer ideas on how to improve the care of a person with Alzheimer's.

H.O.P.E. for the Alzheimer's Journey incorporates a few original emails my brothers and I wrote to one another during this period. They serve to provide information and examples. The emails have been shortened, typos were eliminated, and some names have been removed. Wording may have been added for clarity. The emails are not in chronological order but are appropriate for the theme of the chapter. Below are some milestone dates to allow the reader to understand the particular phase of our journey.

Jan 2003	First email expressing concern
Oct 2003	First attempt to start Alzheimer's medication, Aricept
Apr 2004	Start of Aricept
Sept 2004	Move to assisted living in Ohio, car sold
Oct 2005	Relocation to memory care facility in Delaware
Jan 2006	Start of additional Alzheimer's medication, Namenda
July 2007	Start of low dose anti-anxiety medication (eventually "as needed")
Jan 2014	Approximate start of last stage of Alzheimer's disease
June 2014	Mother passes away

I am opening up the life of my family so *H.O.P.E. for the Alzheimer's Journey* can provide you with insight, tools, and encouragement for your journey. I believe it will make a difference in your life and the life of your loved one. Most of all, I pray my book will be a ray of hope during this season of your life. May it give you hope to become the caregiver you need to be, hope that you can endure the deterioration of your loved one's mind and body, hope that you can take care of yourself, and hope that you can connect with and enjoy your loved one.

I lost my mother, friend, and role model on June 15, 2014. I was blessed to have her with me all of these years. I am grateful for the precious memories we created as her mind and body slowly deteriorated. I am grateful for God's presence throughout. I am grateful for the support of family, friends, and medical and caregiving professionals. I am grateful I was able to help provide the care and quality of life she deserved.

Part I

Preparation for the Alzheimer's Journey

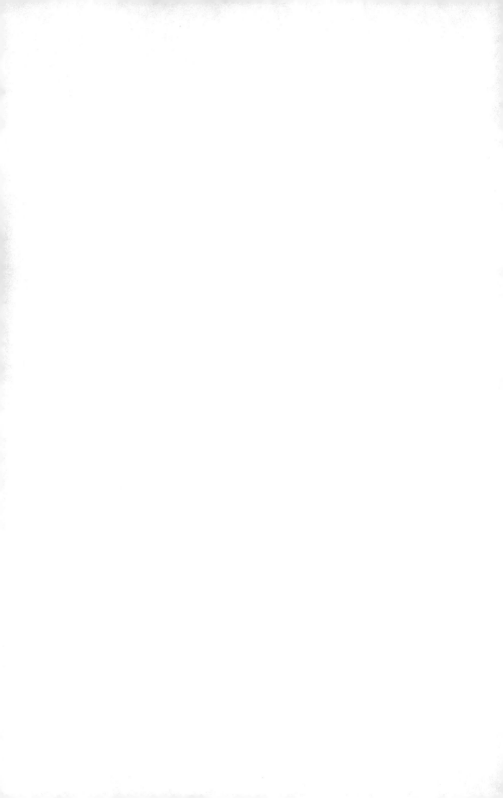

Chapter 1

The Challenge of Caring for a Person with Alzheimer's Disease

• • • •

The biggest challenge of caring for a person with Alzheimer's is to remain hopeful. It was scary knowing my mother had a terminal illness. It was devastating knowing Mom would suffer and deteriorate for years. It was incomprehensible, knowing Mom could forget who I was. I needed hope that I could endure watching my mother waste away from this debilitating disease. I needed hope that I could continue to connect with and enjoy her. I needed hope that researchers would find a cure before it was too late for Mom. I needed hope that I could be the caregiver and daughter she needed in these remaining years of her life. I had to make the most of her last years in spite of the bleak situation. I learned to look for, appreciate, and savor God's rays of hope.

Every sixty-six seconds someone in America develops Alzheimer's disease. There are five-and-a-half million Americans with the disease and more than fifteen million unpaid caregivers for those with Alzheimer's and other dementias. These caregivers provide 18.2 billion hours of care annually[1]. These family members and friends are thrust into their role by necessity, with very little preparation or understanding of how the disease would slowly cause their loved one to deteriorate. I was one of these caregivers for more than eleven years. I was forced to learn how to become a better caregiver so I could provide the care my mother needed and deserved.

Caring for someone with Alzheimer's is difficult because the person's behavior is often different and uncharacteristic. My mother was previously optimistic, but the illness initially made her negative toward situations and persons close to her. Her judgment and behavior became unpredictable. On two consecutive days the reaction to the same situation was completely different. She began to speak what she used to only think. For example, if someone walked by who looked different (defined however you like), I was afraid my mother may say something to embarrass the person…or me.

I remember when my father was dying of cancer I kept telling myself this was not how I would remember him. I was there for my father in those last days, but in the back of my mind I focused on the pleasant memories. I found myself using a similar technique with my mother when she moved to Delaware. I thought of my mother as "she" and "her" and "mother," but not "Mom," "The Mom," or "my Mom." Realizing that slowly, in a way, I was distancing myself from my mother was crucial to reestablishing a more rewarding relationship. I could not keep her at arm's length. Throughout our lives our mother supported my brothers and me 110 percent; I wanted to do the same for her. I am so glad I embraced Mom and the Alzheimer's disease. I have so many precious memories from our time in Delaware I will treasure for the rest of my life. I could not imagine her on the Alzheimer's journey without my 110 percent support. I had to find "my Mom" that was hiding inside. I may not have liked her behavior, but she was still "my Mom." She may have said the wrong thing, but she was "my Mom."

Some days I dreaded going to visit. It was usually when I had to take her to a medical appointment and I could not anticipate her mood or behavior. I usually assumed I would encounter the worst case scenario, which did not help. I should have hoped for the best. I believe she could sense my mood even if I tried to hide it with my behavior. But eventually, on many days, I could visit Mom and truly enjoy her company, quick wit, and sense of humor.

Once when taking Mom to the doctor, the hymn "All Hail the Power of Jesus' Name" was playing on the radio. I reflected on my childhood when my mother decided to teach me church hymns. "All Hail the Power" was one of the first songs she taught me. While listening to the radio and without saying a word to her, I felt a powerful connection to our past and to our present.

Caring for a person with Alzheimer's is difficult because the person has poor short-term memory and eventually begins to lose long-term memory. Memory loss that interferes with the daily routine can be devastating. A person's memory is tied to who they were, who they are, and what they are doing. If a person is sitting in a car without short-term memory, he or she will not know if he or she should get out of the car or buckle his or her seat belt. Initially, Mom only exhibited poor short-term memory, but eventually her long-term memory began to slowly disappear. It was difficult having a basic conversation on many subjects in the past. I learned to incorporate what had happened and what was going to happen in my regular conversations to remind her.

Caring for a person with Alzheimer's is also difficult because someone must take charge of the situation when the person is unable to manage his or her affairs. The person taking charge may be a spouse, sibling, child, other family member, or friend. Taking responsibility for another adult is difficult. Becoming a parent to one's own parent is especially hard when the adult child has probably relied on the parent most of his or her life for guidance, wisdom, and support. Also, the good and bad relationship issues that existed before the diagnosis may remain as responsibility is assumed for the other person. And somehow a loved one may remember what buttons to push to get what he or she wants.

Pride may prevent a person with Alzheimer's from asking for and accepting help. Caregivers must provide care in a way that maintains the dignity of the person. I had to learn how to be a "parent" to my mother without treating her like a child and while continuing to respect her. Early on, before assuming responsibility for our mother, a water pipe burst while she was out of the house. The six-month period of helping her with the home repairs demonstrated my brothers and I had her best interest in mind and increased our credibility with her. This period made it easier for Mom to accept help and the decisions we made on her behalf.

Caregiver situations each have their unique challenges. Some caregivers are caring for a spouse or for multiple parents, one with and one without Alzheimer's. Some caregivers are married, working, and raising children. I was married to Alvin and worked in managerial roles that required travel. I had to balance my time and responsibilities.

Caring for a person with Alzheimer's is also difficult because it takes a physical and emotional toll on the caregiver. In the early phase of our mother's disease, my brother Mike used the phrase, "It's not her fault she has Alzheimer's disease." This phrase was a reminder for my brothers and me to:

- Treat Mom with dignity and respect.
- Not take out our frustrations on Mom.
- Not take Mom's personal attacks personally.
- Not blame Mom for doing what she should not do.
- Not blame Mom for not doing what she should do.
- Pause before reacting to Mom's behavior.
- Have patience, patience, patience.

Caregivers must exhibit a lot of self-control.

Caregivers should do a self-analysis and determine what traits or skills can help and what traits or skills can hinder them from being a good caregiver. My project engineer training helped me as a caregiver. I managed multiple activities simultaneously and systematically worked through issues and barriers. But these same skills hindered me because sometimes I became impatient in wanting to get the job done. I was thankful I had an internal alarm that at times alerted me that I was losing patience. But caregivers can only do the best they can do.

While driving to my mother's, I often asked God for help to deal with any situation that arose. I sometimes used separation to prevent me from being impatient with her. When I visited and she was in a state of extreme agitation and/or confusion, I told myself, "Carol, you can leave in fifteen minutes." Knowing I only had to be patient for fifteen minutes helped to modify my mindset, and many times I remained longer. I knew I could probably ease Mom's state of agitation or confusion.

Sometimes separation was not as easy. In 2011, after a routine doctor's appointment, a blood test was required. I was told the hospital outpatient laboratory closed at 5:30 p.m., but it actually closed at 5 p.m. The hospital graciously arranged to do the blood work, but it took time to work out the details. I was pushing Mom in a hospital wheelchair with her walker hanging across the back handles. She kept repeating, "Why don't we make an appointment and come back?" The blood test could have been done the next day, but it was easier to add the blood work after the doctor's appointment rather than to take her out the next day. Taking Mom to a doctor's appointment created a lot of anxiety for her. Also, I needed to work the next day since I was unable to return to work that afternoon. I was tired and Mom was tired, so I moved her to the waiting area while I completed the paperwork with the emergency room staff. I knew my patience was gone and I did not want to say the wrong thing to my mother.

When my brothers and I started this journey, caring for a person with Alzheimer's was further complicated because we were unaware of a roadmap. We had a guide of seven stages that provided a general idea of how the abilities of a person with Alzheimer's changed as the disease progressed (appendix 1). The caregiver must monitor changes in mood and behavior and work with a doctor to decide if a change in routine, medication, or care is needed.

Throughout this journey I learned to find God's blessings, the rays of hope. I was hopeful when Mom had no pressing medical, housing, or behavioral issues. I was hopeful when I could say the right words and have the right demeanor and gestures to diffuse or prevent a negative situation. I was hopeful when a stranger (angel) offered to help Mom or me. I was hopeful when I could be patient and focus on the needs of my mother. I was hopeful when Mom and the residents were enjoying an evening social. I was hopeful when Mom was using sound logic or showed an increased awareness of her surroundings. I was hopeful when my mother said, "It's eighty degrees," as she correctly read the thermometer dial while exiting the building. I was hopeful when my mother complimented me on my new suit and it was a new suit. I was hopeful when we opened the door to her room and she was ready and knew she was going somewhere.

To: Mike, Ron   Date: 12/27/10
From: Carol   Subject: Christmas

Mom came to our house for dinner. We did have a small miracle. Alvin picked her up and as he passed one of my company's sites, he told Mom that I worked for the company, but at a different location. Mom said, "I know. She works downtown." Alvin almost drove off the bridge. (smile)

God's rays of hope lifted my spirits and strengthened my belief. I began to believe my mother would be relatively well when I walked into her room. I began to believe she would have more good days ahead than tough days. I began to believe her remaining days would allow her to live in peace with dignity.

These challenges make caring for a person with Alzheimer's very difficult. You will have times when you will want to walk away from it all. And sometimes you have to, even just for a short period, to regroup. Understand you are not alone and there is help. The Alzheimer's Association, education on the disease, concepts from this book, and support from family, friends, and other resources can equip you with help and hope for your journey.

CHECKLIST

_____ Strengthen your trust and credibility with your loved one.

_____ Conduct a self-assessment of the traits and skills that can aid and hinder you from being a good caregiver.

_____ Think about who and what support you will need during the tough phases of this Alzheimer's journey.

Chapter 2

Circle of Support

• • • •

*As children, my oldest brother, Ron, was in charge when my
parents left the house. Ron used his authority to direct Mike and
me to clean up and put away our toys to gain favor from our
mother. He was usually the sibling in trouble with our parents so
I often rebelled against his authority. After my parents returned
and heard of the altercation, Mom would say, "We won't always
be around, and someday you will have to look after each other."
Mom was preparing us for the time when we had to depend on
each other for strength and encouragement.*

I was truly blessed to have a brother on each of my arms for most of
this journey. I am grateful that our successes collectively strengthened
us and provided a hopeful outlook for the next crisis that arose.
Ron and I were eight years apart. Ron completed his accounting degree
with a specialty in taxes. He was a great resource for our family's tax
and financial questions. Ron passed away two years before Mom. Mike
and I are five years apart. Mike has a bachelor's and a master's degree in
chemical engineering. He helped cultivate my interest in engineering.
My brothers and I regularly kept in touch although we lived a great

distance apart, Ron in Los Angeles, Mike in Cincinnati, and I in Wilmington, Delaware.

It was natural for the three of us to unite when Mom began to exhibit signs of memory loss. We were different persons with different perspectives, but the same objective, which was to provide excellent care for our mother. My brothers were the foundation of my circle of support. We worked extremely well together and made all decisions jointly. None of us had knowledge in this area, so we spent a lot of time making our decisions. We conducted research, spoke to others, and engaged in discussions. We often solicited input from Mom to understand her wishes and her concerns. When we collectively made a decision, we each supported the decision 100 percent. Our agreement was important to provide a consistent message to our mother.

Mike is an excellent planner and is very detail oriented. He navigated the paperwork (bills, insurance, social security, taxes), visited regularly, and took Mom to many of her medical appointments. Ron visited from California once or twice a year. He routinely provided practical and technical information about our mother's different medical conditions. He conducted most of our Internet and telephone-based investigations, such as identifying a moving company. In my opinion, Ron was more attuned to Mom's thoughts and feelings than Mike and I. His innate understanding of our mother was beneficial as we made decisions on her behalf.

My brothers and I found that our roles changed depending on the situation. For instance, when Mom had knee replacement surgery, each of us provided care for her for a week with a day or two of overlap. I was with Mom for the pre-surgery preparation, surgery, and transfer to the rehabilitation center. Ron was with Mom for the remainder of her rehabilitation center stay and return to her assisted-living facility. Mike took the final stage, which was to facilitate Mom's transition to assisted living and continue her rehabilitation. One sibling usually executed the plan, and the other siblings were available as issues arose.

In 2005 Mom moved to a memory care facility near me in Delaware to receive twenty-four-hour professional care. I provided most of the routine non-professional caregiving, which involved:

- Supplementing her daily care
- Visiting my mother
- Maintaining her contact with the outside world including social outings
- Interacting with the staff
- Arranging for medical care (appointments, medications, etc.)
- Supplying clothing, toiletries, magazines, and other items

This new responsibility required me to balance family, work, and caregiving.

When my brothers visited, we informally discussed Mom's condition and her care. They were in an ideal position to detect changes in our mother because they did not see her as regularly as I did. They brought fresh eyes to the situation and offered ideas or suggestions. This regular assessment of caregiving, with input from her facility staff, enabled us to provide very good care for Mom.

My other immediate family members, my husband, Alvin, Mike's wife, Judy, and their daughter, Moriah, were an important part of this journey. They were not involved in the decision-making, but they were directly affected by our decisions. They experienced the emergency calls, assumed our household duties, and patiently dealt with the constant calls from the siblings or our mother. They were hopeful and lifted our spirits when we were sad or afraid. They have endured our time away from home and our being distracted with Mom's affairs while at home. It was a difficult balancing act, and I must admit I did not always find the correct balance. So I must publicly thank Alvin, Judy, and Moriah for their understanding, support, and love.

Family members are an extremely important resource to anyone starting this Alzheimer's journey. Start discussions with immediate family members early on. Do not limit yourself to family living in the area. Distant family members can support in other ways. Encourage immediate family members who have not seen your loved one recently to visit and observe him or her.

If you sense resistance from family members, try to determine the root cause of the issue. Some causes to consider are:

- Relationships. Your family member may not get along with you, your loved one, or other immediate family members. One of my friends had a poor relationship with her mother, but she cared for her mother because it was the right thing to do. Maybe sibling rivalry is an issue. Initiate one-on-one discussions to begin to understand. Consider getting someone you all trust to help work through the issues.
- Not all family members will be willing or able to support (money, time, etc.) your loved one in the way you believe they should. Discuss the potential consequences of not providing proper care. Accept what they offer within their constraints. With time, they may be able to provide more support.
- Family members may be receiving financial support (loans), housing, or services (babysitting) from your loved one that could be interrupted if other family members are involved. Try to understand what is taking place and how to eventually eliminate this support if appropriate.
- Family members may be in denial that their loved one may have Alzheimer's. They may not have first-hand experience with the incidents you have witnessed. Or they may dismiss these

incidents as unimportant. Allow time for others to understand and accept the situation. They may never accept the situation but continue to interact with the family members and update them on your loved one's condition.

Whatever the issue, try to resolve it as soon as possible. A 2014 Alzheimer's Association poll indicated that 41 percent of Alzheimer's and other dementia caregivers did not have the help of another unpaid caregiver[1]. Try not to be the only person involved with your loved one's care. The family member's help, input, and insight can help you make the best decisions for your loved one. Or consider a close friend who can become part of your circle of support as a resource for important decisions.

Caregivers should seek help from friends and other family members. Often siblings and friends of the person are elderly, may not drive, and may have health challenges. Other family members and friends may be unable to make a regular or long-term commitment. Sometimes people are reluctant to help because they are afraid of saying or doing the wrong thing. They may, however, be willing to do tasks such as picking up a prescription, going to the grocery store, or providing a meal. Develop a list of tasks people can assist with, but be willing to accept whatever help is offered. Even a little help can make a difference. Give your helpers the information they need to be successful. For instance, if someone offers to sit with your father during his ninety-minute nap, give adequate instruction. "If he wakes up early he likes a glass of apple juice, and he likes to watch the travel channel."

My brothers and I received valuable support from our mother's close friends. They provided encouragement and advice while moving our mother to assisted living. They knew her well, understood her concerns, and spoke for her. One friend told me our mother wanted Mike to manage her finances rather than me. I could have easily become upset, but we eased our mother's concern by stating Mike would manage her finances. Our mother's friends faithfully kept in touch by calling and sending her cards, newspaper articles, and church bulletins.

Our large extended family was supportive of our mother especially when she lived alone in Cleveland. They took her to social events, helped her with household issues, and took care of her during an electrical blackout. One of her sisters in Cleveland visited her weekly. Other relatives called and sent gifts and cards with pictures of their family. I told her relatives and friends the cards were recycled. When I saw a card on her dresser I picked it up and said, "What a lovely card from ___." Then I handed Mom the card, and she (or I) read the card aloud again as if she had just received it. And she smiled all over again.

Caregivers should surround themselves with a circle of support to ease the caregiving load. Immediate family, extended family, and friends can provide physical, emotional, and spiritual support during this difficult period. The circle of support can make the journey less stressful and more rewarding.

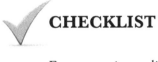 **CHECKLIST**

_____ Encourage immediate family members who have not seen your loved one recently to visit and observe him or her.

_____ Start discussions with immediate family regarding your concerns.

_____ Start discussing your loved one's wishes regarding his or her care and affairs with appropriate family members.

_____ Reassign tasks as the circle of support changes.

Chapter 3

A Watchful Eye

• • • •

The first email in this chapter started our family on this journey.
I became emotional when I re-read it five years later, knowing
what had actually transpired since then.

F amily members should observe their older relatives to make sure they are able to take care of themselves. If you see problems, assess the situation and take necessary action. Beginning in 1999, my brothers and I observed incidents that indicated our mother might not be able to manage as well. We probably missed many more "red flags" because we were not present to observe. By 2002 we were seeing multiple warning signs of her memory loss and lack of comprehension. I sent this email to my brothers on Mom's birthday.

To: Ron, Mike   Date: 1/15/03

From: Carol   Subject: Mom's Birthday

Today is Mom's 83rd birthday. Praise the Lord!

We're at a point where we need to keep a watchful eye on her. It would be good if we can each call her at least once a week to check in. Sometimes it will be a quick call because she will be too busy to talk, and sometimes it will be a long call. The purpose of our calls is to ensure she is all right and not dealing with problems we can assist with.

She went to the doctor after the holidays, and the doctor told her she was worn out. She worked too much before and during our visit. She is as thin as a rail. She was watching her fat intake to lower her cholesterol, but now the doctor is saying to focus on gaining weight. He is also having her take a nap during the day. Personally, I don't know what occupies her time all day. I don't think she manages her personal time as well as she could.

Mom is ok handling the regular day-to-day responsibilities like shopping, groceries, paying bills, etc. Her long-term memory is fading (normal for her age), but she's still alert and fairly sharp. She needs help with non-routine items, and I don't know what all of these items are. We may need to plan some visits to assist with non-routine items. Ron, we realize you won't be able to do this as much, but we may plan some type of task when you're there this summer.

These are some things we need to work on. Our conversations with her will help elaborate on the issues. She can implement the solutions, but let's spend the next few months gathering information and then determine the best way to handle our concerns.

- Cash Flow. Mom has money, but because of low interest rates she tied up a lot of money in long-term certificates of deposits. Mike and I have offered to loan/give her money to tide her over, but she wants to remain self-sufficient. Mike, I don't know if you convinced her to let us pay her real estate taxes. Mike and Judy gave her a restaurant gift certificate, and I sent her one for her birthday. She called the gift certificate a "great pick-me-up." Something is wrong when a $25 buffet restaurant gift certificate is a "great pick-me-up."

- Information. She sometimes misprocesses or misunderstands information. Then she'll worry (which isn't good for her health) for days without calling one of us. Two recent examples:
  - › Her long-term care insurance company was in a class action suit for not informing policyholders of the increased cost for paying in installments. The long-term care insurance company lost and sent Mom information on the settlement. She thought the settlement was remuneration for cancelling her policy. So she spent days thinking her policy was cancelled. During a routine call I explained the situation to ease her mind. Keep in mind what they sent was probably confusing for us to understand.
  - › She is under the impression IRA rules have changed and she can't withdraw her IRA. She believes it's a conspiracy between the IRS and banks to keep the money. I assured her she could withdraw her money. Ron, can you call her regarding this issue?

  Regular calls to Mom can prevent unnecessary worry regarding these kinds of issues.
- House. She mentioned she wanted to do some home repairs. She was not specific, but I said it was a shame she hasn't purchased the carpet yet because she could be enjoying it. We may have to assist her with the process and possibly be there while the work is being done.
- Banking. She's always at the bank, and I don't know why. It makes her more susceptible to robbery or someone getting access to her account. We may need to consolidate her certificates of deposit.

- House Arrangement. Mom is still up and down the stairs in the house. This increases her risk for a fall. We may have to rearrange things to make more room on the first floor. I don't know if she is washing and drying clothes in the basement, but she also has a washer and dryer on the first floor. I don't know if they work. She is also in the basement for food. Maybe a small freezer/refrigerator can fit in the laundry room.

These are the issues we need to think about and gather information. Don't make it obvious we're spying on her because she wants to remain independent. Taking care of some of these issues can help her remain independent. We're really blessed we are dealing with cash flow vs. cash and house vs. nursing home. But we do need to keep a watchful eye on her.

My brothers and I began a period of observing, investigating, collaborating, and careful listening. It was difficult because my brothers and I did not live in Cleveland so we increased our visits and communications. We supplemented our findings by questioning family and friends who saw our mother more frequently about her activities and behavior. We knew we needed to simplify her routine daily activities.

Alzheimer's disease is the most common form of dementia. It accounts for 60 to 80 percent of dementia cases.[1] Alzheimer's is a progressive and fatal disease that gradually damages nerve cells in the brain and the connections between nerve cells. These nerve cells eventually die. Persons with the illness have two abnormal structures in abundance: (1) Amyloid plaques made up of abnormal protein and nerve cell fragments in the memory area of the brain and (2) Neurofibrillary tangles composed of a protein called tau that becomes twisted and interferes with communication within nerve cells. It is not known if these abnormal structures cause or are a product of Alzheimer's disease.[2]

Understanding memory loss was important for us. My brothers and I talked with doctors and with friends in similar situations. We searched the Internet, and each of us visited our local Alzheimer's Association office. The Alzheimer's Association website provides a list of early warning signs. They are:

- Memory loss that disrupts daily life
- Challenges in planning or solving problems
- Difficulty completing familiar tasks at home, at work or at leisure
- Confusion with time or place
- Trouble understanding visual images and spatial relationships
- New problems with words in speaking or writing
- Misplacing things and losing the ability to retrace steps
- Decreased or poor judgment
- Withdrawal from work or social activities
- Changes in mood and personality[3]

Alzheimer's impacts the memory and other cognitive skills such as language, perception, reasoning, judgment, abstract thinking, and attention.[4]

Obtaining an Alzheimer's diagnosis is not easy. A primary care physician can suggest a specialist. The specialist may consult with other specialists (neurologist, psychiatrist, psychologist, etc.). Mom's evaluation included:

- Review of our mother's medical and family history
- A physical exam including chest X-ray, electrocardiogram (EKG)
- Urine and blood tests

- A neurological exam with brain imaging (MRI)
- Tests to check memory and thinking
- Mental health evaluation to rule out depression

People who are heavy snorers or with untreated sleep apnea may have a higher risk of developing memory problems at an earlier age. Sleep apnea is under diagnosed so screening for sleep apnea should be part of the evaluation.[5]

This is an extensive list of tests, but the key is a thorough evaluation to rule out any of the reversible causes of memory loss. The evaluation may pinpoint Alzheimer's as the cause of the memory loss and result in an Alzheimer's diagnosis. But a definitive Alzheimer's diagnosis is not possible until autopsy.[6]

It is important for a person with Alzheimer's to receive a diagnosis and be informed of the diagnosis. Although there is no cure, there are many benefits to an early diagnosis:

- The person can begin treatment with Alzheimer's medication.
- The person can provide input on his or her desires for future care.
- The person can execute legal documents necessary for others to provide care.
- The person can decide on participating in drug trials and be in an early stage of Alzheimer's to increase the chance of acceptance in a trial.

Thirty-two Alzheimer's Disease Research Centers funded by the NIH National Institute on Aging are located in twenty-one states. They can help obtain a diagnosis and provide information, services, and resources. These centers are active in research and coordinate information, research, and data among themselves. A list of these centers can be found on the National Institute on Aging website.[7]

My brothers and I began documenting our mother's symptoms and behaviors. A Cleveland hospital was Mom's medical provider. A geriatric doctor, a specialist who cares for older adults, was her primary care physician. He ensured Mom had completed the screenings and diagnostic testing recommended for an eighty-three-year-old woman. Her doctor was closely monitoring her arthritic left knee, osteoporosis, high cholesterol, and low weight and was aware of her memory loss. He ordered blood tests, memory tests, a baseline MRI, and a neuropsych evaluation specifically to address memory loss. We pieced together much of this information from office reports and appointment schedules for each visit. Mom was receptive to our involvement, and we eventually began taking her to medical appointments and having follow-up communications with her doctors. We were all aware of our mother's memory problems. So we wondered, Why was she not prescribed an Alzheimer's medication?

To: Ron, Mike Date: 9/8/03
From: Carol Subject: Medical

I spoke with the clinic. Mom's neuropsych evaluation summary indicated she did not meet the formal definition for Alzheimer's, but she is at risk for the disease. She is being referred to a community services agency, and a social worker will help assess her needs so she can remain in the house as long as possible. Mom has agreed to this in order to remain in her home. I will follow up with the social worker.

The clinic is also concerned about Mom's weight. She weighs 102 pounds again. We need to remind her to drink two cans of a nutritional supplement daily. Mom gave the clinic permission to share her medical information with me. In recent conversations, Mom appears to be clearer, so maybe the additional sleep is helping. We have to work on the weight.

The neuropsychological evaluation is a combination of interviews, observations, and cognitive testing. Our mother's 2003 report referenced a March 2000 evaluation that identified "diminished working memory" and inefficiencies on "verbal memory tests." The 2000 test findings were "consistent with small vessel disease" (including mini-strokes) rather than Alzheimer's. The 2003 evaluation indicated her difficulty learning a list of unrelated words and her ability to learn and recall stories was borderline-to-average. There was evidence of depression, possibly related to the recent water damage and subsequent home repairs. But she did not meet the clinical requirement for an Alzheimer's diagnosis.

My brothers and I conducted more research on the disease, but we relied on her doctor for the diagnosis. The research helped us develop our questions for the next visit.

To: Carol, Mike   Date: 10/7/03

From: Ron   Subject: (no subject)

Medications on the market do not prevent the disease from getting worse but may slow the decline. Keep in mind that many of the drugs also manage behavioral problems such as hostile behavior, agitation, and other behavioral issues associated with Alzheimer's.[8]

A qualified physician should determine the actual cause of memory loss. So to be diagnosed with Alzheimer's disease, thyroid problems, high blood pressure, hormonal imbalance, anemia, nutritional deficiencies, and infection or pain must be ruled out. These contribute to memory loss and are reversible.[9] Also Parkinson's disease must be ruled out since it may cause memory loss.

Many drugs are on the market, and some of these are new. Closely monitoring and regular reevaluation are very important during treatment with medication.[10]

As I have read over the material, Mom's symptoms do not appear to be at the medication stage, and maybe this is why nothing has been prescribed. She doesn't have the behavioral problems I've seen associated with the illness. I'll send you two the materials I have to date.

Carol, I'm glad you set up this appointment. It's important to know what the doctors have done to rule out any other causes of memory loss and determine if anything can be done at this point to curb the loss.

Activity is recommended which is why the social worker recommended the senior center.

My brothers and I discussed our mother's memory loss with her doctor. Since the doctor diagnosed her as being "at risk" for Alzheimer's, she was not prescribed Aricept. So we were disappointed. We knew if she truly had the disease, the sooner Mom started the medication, the better off she would be. We felt confident the testing was done to exclude other causes of her symptoms. My brothers and I had conducted extensive research on the illness but accepted that we were not medical professionals. Both neuropsych evaluations were based partially on discussions between our mother and the doctor. The reports assumed Mom was telling the truth or could remember when asked if she had difficulties completing daily responsibilities. We knew it was our responsibility to fill the gap. The doctors observed her during a thirty-to sixty-minute visit, but we saw and spoke to Mom regularly. We had to be her advocate so we wrote a follow-up letter to the doctor. We re-iterated our concerns and used the Alzheimer's warning signs to convey examples of further memory loss and confusion.

Our mother's doctors were steadfast that she did not have Alzheimer's but had mild cognitive impairment (MCI)—that is, she was at risk for Alzheimer's. My brothers and I accepted their diagnosis because we had confidence in their capability and reputation. We had a good rapport with her doctors, and they welcomed our involvement. We did not fully agree with the conclusions, but we understood the basis for their decision. Although second opinions can be useful, we decided not to get a second opinion. We focused on increasing our knowledge of our mother's condition and following the doctors' recommendations.

To: Carol, Ron   Date: 11/3/03
From: Mike   Subject: Mini-strokes and Dementia

There is a relationship between mini-strokes and dementia. The following is taken from the book *A Complete Guide: How to Care for Aging Parents* I recently sent to you.

"About 60% of all cases of dementia are the result of Alzheimer's disease. Perhaps 15 to 20 percent are caused by a series of small, often unnoticeable, strokes that produce what is known as multi-infarct dementia, and another 15 to 20 percent are caused by a combination of these two. Less than 10 percent of dementia cases are due to other causes, such as alcoholism, brain damage, and brain tumors, or Creutzfeldt-Jakob, Huntington's, Parkinson's, or Pick's disease."[11]

Mom is on a tightrope with so many medical issues: low weight, low bone density, memory loss, mini-strokes, high cholesterol, etc.

Some of these issues are related. Trying to manage all of this is no easy task for her doctors.

My brothers and I spent the remainder of 2003 hopeful and encouraged Mom to follow the doctors' orders. We worked to increase her weight (ensured she was eating and drinking her nutritional supplement) and to increase her socialization (encouraged her to visit the senior center).

To: Ron, Mike   Date: 12/19/03
From: Carol   Subject: Today

We need to keep the momentum up with the senior center. Mom really liked the "Books and Such" that meets on Tuesday. She obtained a library card and borrowed the book for next week. Today she will try to attend "Stitch Together," ladies who sew, knit, crochet, and cross-stitch, etc. She says she has work to do, so if you talk to her, reinforce the importance of the senior center.

Our mother's Alzheimer's behaviors, such as being suspicious, did increase, however. She believed someone broke into her house and mistakenly accused us of doing things. Her misunderstanding and miscommunications with her bank continued to escalate even though we reiterated that her account had no discrepancies.

To: Carol, Ron
From: Mike

Date: 1/1/04
Subject: Fw: Mom Worried
About Bank Still

The saga continues. To bring Ron up to speed, Carol got a call from Mom this morning regarding the $500 the bank took or is planning to take....

Bottom line. Mom needs help!! If this continues, Mom will not be able to care for herself. The help should originate with her primary doctor. Help could be in the form of psychiatric help, Aricept, home care, assisted living care, or nursing home care. This is serious, and I believe the "wait and see if things get better period" has come to an end.

Please share your thoughts.

To: Carol, Ron
From: Mike

Date: 1/3/04
Subject: Re: (no subject)

Something needs to be done. We need to start with her primary physician and describe the current situation and get her doctor to provide her recommendation. We should be engaged, but none of us are trained to make these calls.

Keep in mind that I believe things have gotten worse. The neurologist's psychiatric treatment approach may be the right next approach, but her geriatric doctor previously disagreed with this approach. I am okay if we want to recommend to the doctor psychiatric treatment for now, but the risk is the window may be closing on Mom having enough memory for Aricept to help retard. We just don't want to wait too late.

The three of us need to agree quickly on the plan and have someone work with the doctor early next week. I suggest Carol contact the doctor since she has been our primary contact with Mom's doctors. I am available to do this with Carol or in her place.

We believe the doctor will support prescribing Aricept because of the escalation of Mom's behavior. If we start with Aricept, we need a system in place to ensure she is taking her medicine and to observe her for side effects.

To: Carol, Mike   Date: 1/5/04

From: Ron   Subject: No Subject

I've read the revised letter to Mom's doctor, and the changes are great. I think the doctors will get the message that there is a problem and the family is asking for assistance. Incidentally, it should be clear this letter, even though sent by Carol, is from all of us and her family is on the same page. I do think Mom's fear of losing her license should be indicated as the reason she cancelled the driving assessment appointment.

Also, I do not think Mom's problems are necessarily a result of memory loss. Driving test, compliance with all of our requests, and bank issues, in my opinion, are Mom's strong desire to remain independent. Unfortunately, this desire is creating other problems. Thus, in discussion of Aricept as an option, I would recommend you discuss Mom's strong desire to remain independent.

A second letter to her doctor outlined further deterioration of our mother's condition. The escalation in behaviors warranted the start of Aricept. Mom did not experience side effects.

To: Ron, Mike   Date: 5/30/04

From: Carol   Subject: Praise the Lord

I spoke to Mom, and she said she is feeling better overall. She said she has been sewing and has the patience to read the instructions and take stitches out if necessary. I've been speaking to her in the evening, and even if she thinks Mike is coming this week, she will correct herself and say he is coming next week for her driver's test. I think the improvement is due to a number of things and not necessarily in this order:

- Getting things done around the house
- Doing some of the things she enjoys, gardening, yard work
- There have been no external major issues.
- Increased socialization, weekly nurse visit, occasional senior center visit, my daily calls, and outings (her neighbor's party, AARP event)
- Aricept

Whether this improvement is real or perceived, it will go a long way for Mom. Keep her in your prayers.

I will arrange a social worker visit after Mom's driving test (just in case).

The Office of Aging invited Mom to a program at the senior center. I will get more information and make sure it is on her calendar and ours so we can remind her.

Our start to this journey was challenging and stressful. My brothers and I did not have a roadmap, and we encountered multiple bumps along the way. The most difficult part was observing a decline in our mother's capability to think, reason, and remember. It was especially hard managing the issues from a distance. Many times Mom was alone and overly concerned with an issue, and we could not say anything to dissipate her concern. Throughout this phase we remained focused as we maneuvered our way through the maze of issues. Our persistence paid off. We felt better after a few successes, a few rays of hope. Mom passed her driving assessment test, and we saw an improvement in her behavior after she started taking Aricept. We continued our communication and had fewer calls of concern and fewer issues. More important, Mom felt she had improved.

Caregivers should seek medical care for loved ones with memory loss. A thorough exam may rule out other causes and narrow the diagnosis to Alzheimer's. Treatment with Alzheimer's medication can slow the progression of the disease and reduce some of the symptoms.

 CHECKLIST

_____ Recognize the Alzheimer's disease early warning signs. If your loved one exhibits these behaviors, have him or her evaluated.

_____ Ensure that your loved one receives regular medical care and is current on medical screenings. If possible, take him or her to the next doctor's visit.

_____ Assess the capability and the living situation of your loved one by having a watchful eye. Help to simplify his or her responsibilities.

_____ Address concerns (safety, health, or financial) with your loved one and appropriate immediate family members.

Chapter 4

The Caregiving Principle™

• • • •

A good relationship with our mother was vital to our success as caregivers. As we interacted with her, however, some difficult situations arose. I wanted to prevent these difficult times from recurring. As I reflected on our mother, these situations, and our caregiving, I developed The Caregiving Principle™. The fundamentals of The Caregiving Principle™ provided additional insight into Mom and helped improve our interactions.

My father passed away in 1987, and our mother adjusted to living alone after forty-one years of marriage. She learned how to maintain her home because she planned to remain in her house as long as possible. My brothers and I visited most holidays. We provided some level of caregiving to Mom the last fourteen years of her life. Initially, the assistance was advice on minor issues such as insurance or selecting a home phone carrier. As our mother's illness progressed, she required more help from family and professional caregivers. The progression of the caregiving she received is shown in table 1.

Table 1 illustrates that the amount of caregiving required is related to the needs of the person and his or her capability. This fundamental concept is called The Caregiving Principle™.

Needs of the Person
minus
Needs Filled by the Person
equals
Needs to Be Filled by the Caregiver(s)

or

Needs of the Person – Needs Filled by the Person =
Needs to Be Filled by the Caregiver(s).

Simply, if a person cannot provide for all of his or her own needs, then someone else must provide them. The "someone else" is a caregiver. For example, apply the principle to a baby and think about how caregiving changes as the baby becomes a toddler, teenager, and then young adult. The Caregiving Principle™ is used throughout this book to understand caregiving for a person with Alzheimer's but can be used for persons with any debilitating condition.

Table 1

Caregiving History

	Symptoms	Family Caregiving	Professionals
Jan 1990 - Feb 2000	None	Occasional help with minor decisions. 8-12 visits/yr from children.	None
Mar 2000 - May 2002	Memory decline detected from neuropsych evaluation.	Occasional help with minor decisions. 8-12 visits/yr from children. Increased calls from children.	None
June 2002- May 2003	Memory loss that disrupts daily life.	15-20 visits/yr from children. Increased calls from children. Weekly visit from sister.	Consult with social worker.
June 2003- Aug 2004	Memory loss that disrupts daily life. Difficulty planning/solving problems. Difficulty completing familiar tasks. Confusion with time and place. Misplacing things. Further memory decline detected from neuropsyche evaluation (July 2003). Change in mood and personality.	20-25 visits/yr from children. Weekly visit from sister. Calls to social worker and nurse. Assist with finances. Manage medical care. Take to social events.	Consult with social worker. Bi-weekly visits from social worker (Oct. 2003). Weekly visit from nurse (Aug. 2004).

Table 1 (cont.)

Caregiving History

	Symptoms	Family Caregiving	Professionals
Sept 2004 - Sept 2005	Memory loss that disrupts daily life. Difficulty planning/solving problems. Difficulty completing familiar tasks. Confusion with time and place. Misplacing things. Change in mood and personality. Decreased or poor judgment.	20-25 visits/yr from children. Weekly visit from sister. Manage finances and medical care and take to social events. Regular calls to assisted living staff.	Assisted living resident. Personal caregiver at night (Sept. 2005).
Oct 2005 - Dec 2013	Memory loss that disrupts daily life. Difficulty planning/solving problems. Difficulty completing familiar tasks. Confusion with time and place. Misplacing things. Change in mood and personality. Decreased or poor judgment.	~160 visits/yr from children (Lives in same area as Carol). Manage finances and medical care and take to social events. Interact with memory care staff.	Memory care facility resident. Basic care level. Hospitalization (April 2007, Dec. 2008) for pneumonia. Medium care level (April 2012).
Jan 2014 - June 2014	Memory loss that disrupts daily life. Difficulty planning/solving problems. Difficulty completing familiar tasks. Confusion with time and place. Misplacing things. Change in mood and personality. Decreased or poor judgment.	Increased visits from children. Manage finances and medical care. Interact with memory care staff. Interact with hospice care staff.	Memory care facility resident. Hospitalizations (Feb. 2014, Mar. 2014, Apr. 2014) for pneumonia and urinary tract infection. High care level (May 2014). Hospice care (last 4 days).

The Caregiving Principle™ broadly defines the needs of a person, which consists of much more than ensuring that activities of daily living (ADLs), such as bathing, dressing, and eating, are met.[1] American psychologist Abraham Maslow defined needs in a way that encompassed the total being. He believed everyone has five levels of needs (figure 1). A person does not have a desire for a need on the upper part of the pyramid until the needs on the lower part of the pyramid are mostly met. The size of the pyramid section shows the magnitude of the need. For example, a person has a need for food (physiological need) every day but may only have a need for self-actualization once a month, once a year, or possibly never. If stranded on an island, for example, once a source of food and water is identified, attention will shift to the need for safety and health. This concept is known as Maslow's Hierarchy of Needs.

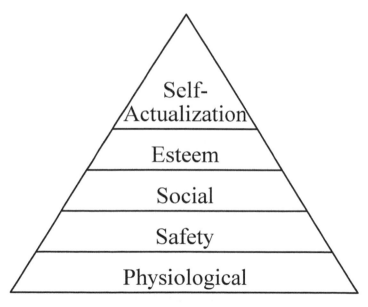

Figure 1[2]
Maslow's Hierarchy of Needs

Based on this concept, the needs of a person are:

- Physiological—air, food, water, and sleep
- Safety—personal security, financial security, health, and well-being
- Social—friendship, intimacy, and family
- Esteem—respect, self-esteem, and need to be accepted and valued by others
- Self-actualization—need to realize one's maximum potential

Evaluating my mother's needs using Maslow's theory helped me understand her much better. I observed her need for all of these levels when she lived in Delaware. To meet a **physiological** need, she kept a glass of water in her room. Overly concerned about how and when she would return, Mom was uncomfortable leaving her facility, which had become a safe and familiar environment and met her need for **safety**. She frequently asked how the family was doing, or if she was in her room she ventured to the living room to see what the other residents and caregivers were doing. She was satisfying her **social** need by hearing family news and interacting with other residents and caregivers.

Sometimes my mother tried to mask her Alzheimer's. Often, in the doctor's waiting room, she whispered to me, "What doctor am I here to see, and what am I here for?" She was trying to maintain her **esteem**. She cared what others thought about her. I once made a comment about the caregivers helping her with a shower, and she replied, "I'm not helpless. I don't need help getting a shower." She wanted to operate at her maximum potential (**self-actualization**) even at a time when her cognitive and physical states were declining.

Maslow states that if the physiological need (air, food, water, and sleep) of a person is not met, the deficiency will have a physical impact on the body (for example, dehydration, constipation). When the safety, social, and esteem needs are not met, the deficiency may affect the mind and behavior. "The body gives no physical indication, but the individual feels anxious and tense."[3]

Anxiety is one of the behaviors exhibited by persons with Alzheimer's.[4] When I reviewed some of the conflicts with my mother, the root cause was her need to meet one of these five needs. I believe many Alzheimer's behaviors, such as anxiety, aggression, suspicion, and hallucinations, can be a result of unfulfilled physiological, safety, social, or esteem needs. To help manage behaviors, the Alzheimer's Association brochure on behaviors advises caregivers to determine if the person's needs are being met.[5] It is hoped that understanding and meeting the physiological, safety, social, or esteem needs of a person can reduce his or her anxiety and some of the behaviors.

Before the diagnosis the person met most if not all of his or her needs independently. Meeting all of the needs of a person with the illness provides a good quality of life. Applying Maslow's Hierarchy of Needs to a person with Alzheimer's may appear to be a daunting task for a family caregiver. In many cases, providing the first two needs (physiological and safety) requires much more than many caregivers can physically and mentally handle. The primary caregiving focus should be providing the lower needs of the pyramid such as eating, bathing, sleeping, health, and safety in a way that maintains his or her esteem. Family members or friends not directly involved with providing care can help meet his or her social or self-actualization need. As the illness progresses, the first two needs (physiological and safety) will require more caregiver time, and the person may show less need or appreciation for the needs on the upper portion of the pyramid. The "Needs of the Person" part of The Caregiving Principle™ is discussed further in Part II.

Applying Maslow's Hierarchy of Needs to my mother was truly eye opening. Alvin brought Mom to our house on Thanksgiving Day, 2009. She enjoyed the fellowship but started to ask some variation of the same question. "How did I get here?" "Is my car parked out front?" The Thanksgiving meal met my mother's **physiological** need. The visit and the interaction with Alvin and me met her **social** need. After dinner I had planned to play Wheel of Fortune because she enjoyed watching the show on television. I wanted to test if the game would be stimulating or frustrating for her. Mom did not want to play. She wanted to return home (memory care facility) because home provided her the **safety** she needed. Until my mother's need for **safety** was fulfilled, she had no desire to fulfill the **social** need. Understanding Mom's need for safety prevented me from being upset. I knew why she wanted to go home, so I took her back and went Christmas shopping afterward. My mother was content, and so was I. Throughout the years my brothers and I had many conflicts with our mother. Understanding Mom's needs could have helped us in many of those early situations.

The second part of The Caregiving Principle™ is "Needs Filled by the Person." These needs are filled based on the capability of the person, as defined by the cognitive capability (which declines as the disease progresses) and the physical ability (which declines with age and as the disease progresses). My family worked proactively to slow the decline of our mother's cognitive capability and physical ability so that she could continue to care for herself. The ability to care for herself, in turn, contributed to my mother's self-esteem. The costs of caregiving are significant, both the financial expense and the toll it takes on family and friends. Reducing caregiving by slowing the cognitive and physical decline of a person with Alzheimer's benefits everyone. Part III discusses the cognitive capability and physical ability of a person with Alzheimer's.

The last part of The Caregiving Principle™ is "Needs to Be Filled by the Caregiver(s)." Caregiving is providing those needs a person cannot provide for himself or herself in a caring and dignified manner. Caregiving can involve one or multiple family, friend, or professional caregivers. For instance, one caregiver may focus on the person, like feeding or bathing, and another caregiver may focus on household support, such as cooking or laundry. If the person resides in a facility, the facility will meet the basic needs, and family members can supplement the care to provide a good quality of life.

The last three sections, Part IV—"Tools for the Caregiver to Fulfill Needs," Part V—"Meeting Needs in Different Residential Settings," and Part VI—"Advice for the Caregiver," focus on equipping caregivers with tools, information, advice, and hope for the Alzheimer's journey.

The Caregiving Principle™ is a simple framework to ensure the needs of the person are met and a good quality of life is provided. It provides caregivers a better understanding of their loved one to make the journey less stressful and more rewarding.

 CHECKLIST

_____ Recall a difficult encounter with your loved one and determine if Maslow's Hierarchy of Needs provides additional insight.

_____ Identify a specific area where The Caregiving Principle™ can help you better care for your loved one.

Part II

The Caregiving Principle™: Needs of a Person with Alzheimer's Disease

Chapter 5

Physiological Need

• • • •

When my mother lived alone, she purchased groceries, cooked, and ate, but her weight continued to drop. She stopped wearing shorts and short sleeves to mask her weight decline. Only a trip to the doctor showed her fragile body. My brothers and I did not understand how dangerously close we were to dealing with more pressing medical issues.

The Caregiving Principle™, introduced in chapter 4, states: **Needs of the Person – Needs Filled by the Person = Needs to Be Filled by the Caregiver(s).** The physiological need is the most important need in the pyramid. Maslow defines the physiological need as the basic needs of the body to survive, such as food, water, sleep, air, and excretion.[1] These basic needs are similar to activities of daily living (ADLs) a set of common, daily tasks needed for personal care and independent living that include transferring, toileting, bathing, dressing, eating, and sleeping. The ability of a person to perform his or her ADLs is used by medical professionals to determine if a person is able to care for himself or herself.[2] Instrumental activities of daily living (IADLs) are tasks that support the ADLs, such as cooking, cleaning, and managing finances.[3] The physiological need, as defined in the Caregiving Principle™, encompasses ADLs, IADLs, and providing shelter.

Activities of Daily Living (ADLs)

Transferring. Transferring is a person's ability to transfer himself or herself in and out of a bed, chair, wheelchair, etc. Persons with Alzheimer's usually lose the ability to walk or transfer during the late stages of the disease.[4] The inability to transfer may be the result of an injury or another illness. Equipment, such as transfer belts or slings, bed cane or rail, seat lifters, and hydraulic body lifts, can help with the transferring process.

To: Carol   Date: 3/10/14

From: Mike   Subject: Re: Monday, 3/10 a.m.

When I returned to the hospital the physical therapist was working with Mom. Mom was sitting on the side of the bed. She was trying to get Mom to stand up. I even helped her try. The therapist tested her legs/knees for pain, and Mom said she had no pain. She then was able to get Mom to stand for just a few seconds before she sat back down on the side of the bed. She believes Mom's problem is not pain but knowing how to get the brain to get the body to stand. It is a processing issue. She plans to see Mom again tomorrow.

Toileting. In the early stages of the disease, persons with Alzheimer's can manage toileting needs. As the disease progresses, however, they may need reminders or prompting to use the bathroom. Eventually they may need help or prompting with wiping, disposing of toilet paper, flushing the toilet, and washing hands. Incontinence is usually only present in the later stages of the disease.[5] Incontinence is not an easy subject to discuss and should be done gently.

Poor short-term memory in the early stage may cause a person not to remember the bathroom location or that he or she has to use the bathroom. Mike and I always had our mother use the restroom before leaving her facility and before returning from our destination. Mom almost always used the bathroom if offered because she did not know when she would have another opportunity. Mike often suggested a bathroom break while they were waiting in a doctor's office to help break up the wait time.

Bathing/Grooming. Bathing an elderly person with Alzheimer's presents many challenges. In the early stages of the disease, he or she can bathe himself or herself, so safety should be the primary concern. Bathing can be dangerous because of wet surfaces, tight spaces, and having to climb into the bathtub or shower. Increase the safety of bathing by installing grab bars and slip-resistant tape and by adding a shower chair. Have everything available and remain with the person while he or she is bathing. Most elderly facilities have showers rather than bathtubs to help reduce falls.

As the disease progresses, the person may be able to bathe but may not choose or remember to do so. He or she may not want to get undressed, lose the privacy, or feel the wet or cold. The goal of the caregiver is to make bathing as pleasurable as possible.[6] Explain what is happening because your loved one may not be accustomed to receiving assistance. Music may set the mood, a space heater can keep the room warm, and large towels or a terrycloth robe can speed up the drying process. Even though my mother had lost her sense of smell, I purchased scented shower gel, which gave her and her room a nice scent. Plus, she received compliments throughout the day, which was also a boost to her self-esteem.

Dressing. In the early stages, persons with Alzheimer's can dress themselves. As the disease progresses, they may begin wearing the same clothing every day. As the disease progresses, they may wear clothes that do not match or clothes inappropriate for the season or time of day. Eventually they will require more help until they are unable to dress themselves.[7]

When my mother moved to assisted living, my mother began wearing the same outfit over and over again. This habit continued when she moved to the memory care facility. One caregiver originally thought Mom only had one or two outfits until she saw her closet. The caregiver took the favorite outfit one night to force Mom to wear something different. The caregivers began to periodically give me a bag of clean clothes Mom wore too often. I took the clean clothes home and rotated them back in her closet one or two months later or the next season.

I bundled my mother's underclothes for each day in small, clear, zippered bags to make it easier for her to get dressed. I labeled each bag "Sunday's underwear," "Monday's underwear," and so on. It was a good idea, but my mother did not use the bundled underwear. One of the caregivers appreciated the bagged items, though, when she helped my mother shower and dress.

I sometimes assisted dressing Mom in her room or at a doctor's office. Sometimes she was unsure if she was dressing or undressing, so I constantly prompted her. I tried not to repeat, "Put your blouse on. Put your jacket on." Instead I would say:

"Looks like you are ready for your blouse."
"Here's your favorite turtleneck."
"This jacket matches the pants you are wearing."
"I'll get your shoes while you are putting on your socks."

I limited my mother's clothing options in memory care to simplify clothes selection in the morning. To simplify dressing, I purchased pants with an adjustable (elastic or drawstring) waist and shoes with a Velcro closing. Persons with the disease often break zippers, so I purchased jackets with large button closures. Pullover sweaters eventually became more difficult for my mother to put on so I started purchasing blouses, turtlenecks with a snap closure, and mock turtleneck sweaters. The daughter of one resident selected her father's clothing so every shirt matched every pair of pants.

I purchased machine-washable and permanent-press clothes for my mother, which allowed the staff to wash them. Some family members will choose to do the laundry of their loved one who lives in a facility.

Eating. Proper hydration and good nutrition are important throughout the disease. In the early stages, persons with Alzheimer's can feed themselves. My brothers and I often took my mother out to dinner when family visited. It provided variety and became another outing. We selected a restaurant she liked with a table away from noise. Noise sometimes agitated or distracted Mom. I suggested an entree my mother liked to remove the pressure of her ordering.

As the disease progresses, the person with Alzheimer's may need prompting to eat. Eating will become very messy. It may be easier to serve finger foods (sandwiches, chicken fingers, French fries). During the latter stages, persons with the disease will have difficulty swallowing. They may put the food in their mouth but not remember to swallow or be unable to swallow, often "pocketing" the food in their cheeks. Persons with difficulty swallowing are at risk of aspiration, breathing food or liquids into the airways or lungs. This can lead to aspiration pneumonia.

Mechanical soft and pureed foods are easier to eat for a person with difficulty swallowing. A mechanical soft meal is a normally cooked and seasoned meal, but one that has been further processed with a blender, grinder, or knife. The food requires less chewing and is easier to swallow.

During my mother's 2014 rehabilitation stay, the caregiver removed the cover from the mechanical soft dinner prescribed by her doctor. Mom gave me a look that said, "You can do better than this." Mechanical soft meals are visually unappealing, and Mom was anticipating a more appealing meal.

To: Mike   Date: 4/15/14

From: Carol   Subject: Mechanical soft diet

I am at the hospital with Mom. She is in a chair eating. She has mashed potatoes, green beans (not cut up), chicken (1/4-3/4" fine pieces) and thickened fruit juice.

Sleeping. In the early stages of the disease, persons with Alzheimer's will sleep through the night. As the disease progresses, they will often have a disruption to the sleep cycle and eventually confuse night and day. This phenomenon is known as sundowning. Sundowning is late-day (as the **sun** begins to go **down**) confusion, anxiety, and agitation. It may be a result of exhaustion, lighting changes, the need for less sleep, disorientation from dreams, or an upset of one's "internal body clock."[8] This disruption can destroy the routine of a person with the illness.

My mother did not receive adequate rest in the early stages of her disease. She did not have enough hours to accomplish what she needed probably because of unproductive hours. She often went to bed late and got up early. She also adopted the habit of doing tasks when she thought about them because she was afraid she would forget.

In assisted living, my mother eventually started going to the lobby in the evening to make sure the doors were locked. The frequency and lateness of these trips increased and prevented her from getting adequate rest. In memory care, her confusion with night and day began when she decided not to have dinner. She would go to sleep and later that night awake and go to the kitchen thinking it was morning. The staff served her the dinner they had saved for her, and she watched television afterward. It is important to have a safe environment during these late hours.

A hospital bed was prescribed for my mother to elevate her head. The bed also helped with transferring since the bed could be raised to help her get up and helped with safety since it could be lowered to reduce the impact of a fall.

To: Carol   Date: 5/10/13

From: Mike   Subject: Home Hospital Beds

I found the following on the Internet.

"Does Medicare Cover Hospital Beds?

Medicare will cover a hospital bed when you can show a medical necessity for the bed. You must also be covered under Medicare Part B. The doctor must document your need in your medical records and write you an order (prescription) for the equipment. Do not order anything until you have a doctor's prescription no matter what the salesperson tells you. The supplier must receive the order before Medicare is billed, and it must be kept on file by the supplier."[9]

Instrumental Activities of Daily Living (IADLs)

Individuals may be able to perform their ADLs, but to be truly independent they need to be able to go shopping, launder clothes, cook, clean, and handle finances. Tasks that support the ADLs are called instrumental activities of daily living (IADLs). Table 2 displays a list of activities (including IADLs) needed to support ADLs.

Table 2
IADLs and Activities to Support ADLs

ADLs	IADLs and Activities to Support ADLs
Multiple	Maintain household Secure and use transportation Use telephone Manage finances (banking, pay bills, etc.) Use appliances (stove, washer, dryer, etc.)
Transferring	Secure and maintain wheelchair, walker, cane, etc.
Toileting	Purchase products for toileting Use incontinence products
Bathing	Purchase products for bathing Launder towels
Dressing	Purchase clothing Launder clothing
Eating	Purchase groceries Prepare meals Wash dishes
Sleep	Purchase linen Change and launder linen

The failure, inability, or poor quality in which a person performs his or her IADLs is usually an indicator that the loved one is having difficulty with memory. IADLs require memory, reasoning, and judgment skills that are declining in a person in the early stages of Alzheimer's disease. Here are some indicators to watch for:

- Late bill notices
- Utilities shut off
- Bounced checks
- Checks not recorded in checkbook
- Unbalanced checkbook
- Leaving doors unlocked
- More than usual clutter
- Odors in the home
- Trouble using appliances
- Leaving water running
- Leaving lights on
- Clothes in disrepair
- Poorly fitting clothes
- Laundry piling up
- Too many groceries
- Leaving ingredients out of food
- Burning food
- Leaving stove burners on
- Not taking medication
- Arriving places (appointments, church, etc.) on wrong day/time
- Getting lost going to a familiar place

These indicators should be compared with how the person performed these tasks prior to the onset of the disease.

There are many ways to assist a person with IADLs. Meals on Wheels, bank direct deposit of income checks, automatic bill pay, mail-order pharmacy, and delivery services of grocery stores and pharmacies can help maintain the independence of someone in the early stages of Alzheimer's. The primary question is: should this person be left or live alone?

My brothers and I took an active role in helping our mother with IADLs, such as household and financial issues, as her cognitive capability declined when she lived alone. Ron suggested we create a checklist, which she sometimes used, to help her manage daily activities.

To: Ron, Mike

From: Carol

Date: 10/2/03

Subject: Checklist Item

The checklist idea is good. We have to think about what should be on the list in two years so I've added a few things. Maybe have two lists (morning and night) on a two-sided laminated sheet. Make three copies, one for the bedroom, one for the kitchen, and one extra.

Morning

___Adjust heat or air conditioning

___Take medication

___Take osteoporosis medication on Wednesday

___Drink nutritional supplement

___Check calendar for medical or other appointments

___Plan the day's activities (trip to senior center, nap)

Night

___Review tomorrow's activities, appointments

___Check that garage door is closed

___Check that screens and doors are locked

___Make sure the stove and oven are off

___Make sure lights are out in the basement and second floor

___Drink nutritional supplement

Eating was the primary physiological need my brothers and I were concerned about when our mother lived alone. Mom lost a lot of weight. We started giving her restaurant gift certificates. Her routine was to arrive at her favorite buffet restaurant in the late afternoon, pay the lunchtime price, and start selecting her food as the restaurant transitioned to the dinner menu. Mom often found ways to stretch her dollar.

Caregivers may need to assist with meeting the ADLs and IADLs of a loved one. As the disease progresses, the caregivers will need to provide additional help with both. Caregivers should seek additional help (family, friends, or professionals) to reduce stress and ensure that the physiological need is met.

✓ CHECKLIST

_____ Evaluate the capability of your loved one to perform his or her ADLs and IADLs.

_____ Determine how others (family, friends, community organizations, professional caregivers) can support your loved one with his or her ADLs and IADLs.

_____ Determine if your loved one should be left alone or even live alone.

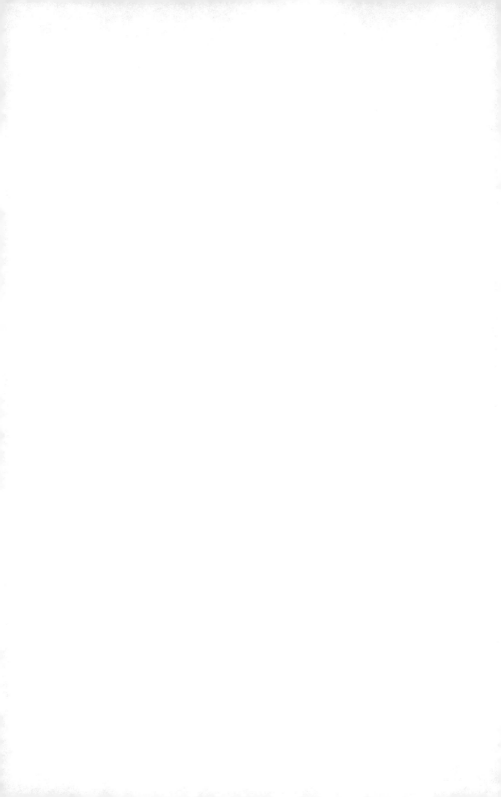

Chapter 6

Safety Need

• • • •

My mother religiously visited the sick and the shut-in members from her church in their homes, their children's homes, hospitals, and nursing homes. I believe these visits prompted her to contemplate her later years. My father died in 1987, and in 1991 my mother purchased a long-term care insurance policy with a second policy in 1997. She read a lot and never wanted to be a burden.

The safety need is the second most important in the pyramid of needs. The need for safety includes physical safety at home and away, a sense of security, financial security, and good health.[1] Good health is discussed in chapter 11, Physical Ability.

Physical Safety

An elderly person may feel safe and secure at home but have unsafe routines and live in an unsafe environment. Safety should be the first concern family members address for the elderly. A person with Alzheimer's is at increased risk for injury because of lack of judgment, and this risk increases as the disease progresses.

Elderly women are susceptible to falling and breaking bones. Twenty to 30 percent of the elderly who break a hip will not live longer than one year. Of those who do survive, many will have significant functional loss. Ninety percent will be unable to climb five stairs after a year even though they needed no help before the fracture.[2] Those with Alzheimer's disease have a greater risk of falling because of balance and gait disorders caused by visual and spatial perception due to the disease. Falls by older adults with a low risk for falls may be an early warning sign of Alzheimer's.[3]

My brothers and I walked through, identified, and corrected unsafe situations in our mother's home. We reviewed her routines and tried to minimize unsafe behaviors. Many of our safety improvements were geared to reducing the risk of a fall because Mom was frequently using the stairs. We tried to consolidate her activities on the main floor.

My brothers and I made the environment safer by:

- Arranging for an emergency response system offered by her local fire department
- Installing handrails on the stairs to the basement and second floor
- Installing safety bars in the bath area and an elevated toilet seat
- Installing additional night lights
- Repairing her first floor laundry tub so she could do laundry on the first floor
- Purchasing a hip protection device to cushion her in case of a fall
- Purchasing phones and programming for emergency, family, and friends
- Arranging for a neighbor's professional lawn service to mow the lawn and helping with yard work (trimming bushes, fertilizing) when visiting
- Providing a laminated card with phone numbers (cell, home, work) of immediate family, a friend, and social worker
- Providing a daily reminder list

- Providing two digital clocks with a large time, date, and day display
- Insisting our mother complete a driving evaluation
- Installing new outside door locks and informing the police she was a senior citizen living alone

A handyman completed the home upgrades. Mom was very receptive to the changes, but she only wore the hip protector sparingly.

I have since found many helpful ideas to aid the safety of a person. For instance, if they have a cell phone, add a contact named ICE (in case of emergency) and list your phone number. Two excellent resources for safety in the home and away are:

- *Staying Safe: Steps to Take for a Person with Dementia*, Alzheimer's Association[4]
- *Home Safety and Alzheimer's Disease*, United States Department of Health and Human Services, NIH, National Institute on Aging[5]

When should a person stop driving? This is an extremely delicate issue and depends on the person. Elderly drivers want to maintain their independence. Family members fear a mistake such as accelerating rather than braking can cause property damage or personal injury or death to the driver, other drivers, passengers, or pedestrians.

My mother voluntarily stopped driving long distances and reduced her night driving. When I visited her in Cleveland, she picked me up at the rapid transit station. She sometimes asked me to drive home, but I pretended to be tired so I could assess her driving capability. Mild cognitive impairment or Alzheimer's can impact a driver's ability. Driving requires quick judgment and quick reaction time. Drivers must remember how to operate the car, driving laws, where they are, and where they are going. I observed Mom for speed, reflexes, alertness, eye contact, ability to remain in her lane, and overall driving capability. I never observed any major issues, but I encouraged her to use her turn indicators more. She took a seniors' driving course and passed a driving assessment her doctor recommended. This issue was solved when she moved to assisted living and we sold her car.

Persons with Alzheimer's disease are at risk for "wandering." They may leave to go somewhere and become lost. That "somewhere" can be real, imagined, near, or far. They may think they have to go to school or work. I have seen news stories where a person with Alzheimer's had driven hundreds of miles from home. The person was found safe, but this is not always the case. I arrived at Mom's memory care facility one day and found her upset because she could not remember where she left her children. Frantically, she was dialing the phone; if she could have left she would have gone in search of her children. Alzheimer's disease caused the events of her life to be rearranged in her mind.

The Alzheimer's Association offers Medic Alert + Safe Return,[6] a program that supplies identification pendants or bracelets. If a person is missing, a community support network, which includes law enforcement, is engaged to help reunite the person with family members. The Alzheimer's Association sponsors Comfort Zone,[7] a web application to monitor a person's location. Many police departments sponsor Project Lifesaver, an international program aimed at the quick recovery of adults and children who wander. These two programs track missing persons using a signal sent from a tracking device.[8] Delaware issues Gold Alerts (similar to Amber Alerts) to help recover missing senior citizens, persons with disabilities, or persons who are suicidal.[9]

Inform others who come in contact with the person routinely of his or her tendency to wander. Neighbors, the mail carrier, neighborhood businesses, for example, can be a second line of defense. My church family kept an eye on my mother when we were separated at church events. For instance, after a church social, I brought my car to the country club entrance to pick up Mom. A friend, without my asking, waited with her to ensure she did not leave on her own.

Provisions should be made for weather emergencies. Develop a plan in case of evacuation, power outage, or loss of water for an extended period of time.

To: Mike, Ron   Date: 8/27/11

From: Carol   Subject: Shelter-in-Place

Mom's facility called to let us know they are going to shelter-in-place during the storm. They have a generator. They left a corporate number if we can't reach them. I'm going over now to take some extra meds and supplies in case we have to evacuate.

Some persons with mild cognitive impairment (MCI), or who are at risk for Alzheimer's, will eventually develop the dementia.[10] One day the person is suffering from memory loss but exhibits fairly sound judgment. The next day or week the person may be irrational and exhibit poor judgment. This poor judgment can put the person in harm's way. Chapter 19, "I Never Thought She Would…," discusses our family's harrowing event that put our mother in harm's way. Suggestions to prevent similar situations are discussed.

A Sense of Security

Maslow's definition of safety encompasses "freedom from fear, from anxiety and chaos." He suggests children will not feel safe if confronted with some new, unfamiliar, or strange situations.[11] These same situations can make a person with Alzheimer's feel less secure. Routines and familiar people and surroundings provide the sense of security a person with Alzheimer's needs. In fact, the need for this security is crucial.

To meet her need for a sense of security, my mother believed she had to reserve her room daily at her memory care facility. Each afternoon she wrote dated notes to the staff: "Elizabeth staying in Room 26 tonight." I am sure some days she wrote five to ten of these notes. If I or the staff told her she did not have to reserve her room, she became indignant or politely acknowledged the comment and wrote a note anyway. At times early on, I tried to prevent her from writing these notes by not giving her paper or pen. Sometimes I carefully took the paper or pen away. But Mom believed she needed a place to sleep and she was going to do what she thought was necessary to secure a room. After analyzing the situation with an understanding of her needs, I began to support her. These notes reduced my mother's anxiety and increased her perceived sense of security.

My mother felt safe and secure at her memory care facility. As her condition progressed, it became difficult to get her to leave. In May 2010, I planned to take her to our church's Mother's Day Brunch. When I arrived, Mom was ready but did not want to go. The caregiver and I would encourage her and she would stand up, and the next minute she would sit back down. Deep down, I knew my afternoon would be easier if my mother did not attend and I would not be bombarded with her repeated questions. But it was a Mother's Day celebration, and I wanted to spend time with her. She was ninety years old. How many more opportunities would I have to celebrate Mother's Day with her? I knew once she was there, she would feel fairly comfortable in the Christian environment. I tried to address her concern by reassuring her she would return. Mom eventually agreed, and once we were in the car she said, "It's good to get out now and then." I just smiled. And we both enjoyed the brunch.

Financial Security

Financial security is an important part of the need for safety. The elderly have a great need for financial security. They never want to be "a burden on anyone." Chapter 16, Legal Affairs, discusses legal documents to initiate as soon as possible if they do not exist. These documents allow caregivers to manage their loved one's assets.

My mother grew up during the Great Depression, which greatly shaped her views of money. Providing my mother a sense of financial security was difficult, especially when she managed her own affairs. She began to misunderstand financial issues with banks, insurance, pensions, and so on.

To: Ron, Mike   Date: 8/23/04

From: Carol   Subject: Bank

Mom called tonight to tell me her bank is closed. She read to me how the bank was bought out by another bank. She remembered I like to have her read the letter or item of concern so she had Sunday's newspaper in front of her. She then mentioned she didn't know if it was closed or not. So even though she really was not concerned (she knew her money was safe), she felt better after the call.

She likes to talk about the country being in a depression and people being out of jobs, but I always refute that. I told her a lot of people aren't in the bank because they can do online banking.

Elderly persons are susceptible to scam artists and those with Alzheimer's even more so. Caregivers should monitor the mail and phone calls. I placed my mother's phone number on the "Do Not Call" list, which helped, but she often received calls from an automobile warranty salesperson. Since my mother no longer had a car, these calls were disruptive because she then started looking for her car.

Long-term care insurance can help with financial security but has to be purchased prior to signs of memory loss. It pays for in-home care or long- or short-term care at an assisted-living facility, memory care facility, or nursing home. The policies pay a daily rate for a specific period such as $70 a day for three years. Certain rules apply for when a person qualifies for benefits, when benefits start, and what services are covered.[12] Long-term care insurance is expensive and is not a good option for everyone. In general, long-term care insurance is recommended as a safety net for persons with assets between $300,000 and $500,000 (excluding a home).[13] Persons without substantial savings will use Medicaid to cover long-term care costs. People with more than $500,000 in assets can pay long-term care costs from their assets.

My mother did not have the recommended assets, but she felt it was necessary to sacrifice to pay the long-term care insurance premiums. She gave us a big scare when we wanted to initiate claims on the policies.

To: Carol, Ron   Date: 9/6/04
From: Mike   Subject: One Long-Term Care
                              Insurance Policy Cancelled?

Tonight Mom said she dropped one of her long-term care insurance policies this year because it was becoming too expensive ($5,000 per year) and her money was running short. Is that true? I thought you had a system in place where if she missed a payment, the insurance company would contact you.

Can you check to see if she currently has both policies in force? She paid on one of the policies, which cleared the bank on 9/3/04, and the next withdrawal put her in the negative. Hopefully, she is mixed up from when they went from semi-annual payments to annual payments.

To: Ron, Mike   Date: 9/8/04
From: Carol   Subject: Both LTC policies valid
Both policies are valid.
   Policy 1 $70/day for three years ~ $1500/year premium
   Policy 2 $60/day for four years ~ $2400/year premium

My mother's long-term care policy provided options when she could no longer live alone. Since she was still quite active, we believed the residents, environment, activities, and outings in assisted living offered a better quality of life than a nursing home. While living in assisted living, the policies did not pay the full daily claim rate so the policies lasted longer. We did not want our mother concerned about her finances, so we always told her the insurance covered everything, even after the policies were depleted.

My brothers and I had to monitor her finances. When she moved to Delaware, I created a ten-year projection of her savings, income, and expenses. I assumed her facility expenses would increase 3 percent annually based on the three-year average Social Security cost-of-living adjustment. I estimated that her care level (and cost) would increase every two to three years due to deterioration from the illness. This projection was updated with actuals and helped us predict when she would run out of money. We developed scenarios for what we would do when that happened based on her cognitive and physical condition.

If she could enjoy the benefits of her memory care facility, we would probably find the money to pay for it. We considered moving her from her shared suite to a double room to extend her money, but we decided against it because the transition in the late stages of the disease would be extremely disruptive.

Mom was always concerned about money. When she went on outings, the activity director often told my mother the outing was free or they used coupons so my mother would not be concerned with the cost. Once my mother knew how the bill would be paid she could enjoy the outing.

The safety need encompasses physical safety, having a sense of security, financial security, and good health. Develop a physical safety plan to keep loved ones from falling, wandering, getting injured, or driving when they should not. A familiar living environment gives the loved one a sense of security which is critical for comfort and to minimize anxiety. Develop a financial plan for the financial security of the loved one and the caregiver.

✓ CHECKLIST

_____ Obtain the two recommended safety resources to ensure a safe physical environment for your loved one.

_____ Consider an emergency response system especially if your loved one lives alone.

_____ Perform a driving assessment if appropriate.

_____ Enroll your loved one in Medic Alert + Safe Return sponsored by the Alzheimer's Association if appropriate.

_____ Recognize the importance of the sense of security for persons with Alzheimer's.

_____ Understand the financial health of your loved one (assets, debts, income, expenses, insurance, etc.).

Chapter 7

Social Need

• • • •

In 2006 I took my mother to the annual show of a skating club. She had always loved figure skating on television. The day after the event she kept telling her caregiver how much she enjoyed it. My mother did not always remember our outings, but I made sure she enjoyed herself at the time. My mother taught me to live in the moment.

The social need, the third need in the pyramid, is the need for belonging, love, and affection. If this need is not met, the person will experience feelings of alienation, strangeness, and loneliness.[1]

Periodically scheduling a social outing, even with another family member or friend helps fill the social need and improves the quality of life for a person with Alzheimer's. Take advantage of times when not many issues are pressing. Social opportunities often create a time when the loved one remembers engaging in similar activities earlier in his or her life. Persons in your circle of support can call, visit, take the person for a ride, or have the person help with a project (plant flowers, fix faucet, etc.).

Caring for a spouse with Alzheimer's has social challenges for both spouses. A better understanding of spousal relationships can be found on the "Changes to Your Relationship" section of the Alzheimer's Association website.[2]

My brothers and I tried to maintain Mom's quality of life while she lived alone in Cleveland. She continued her work at church, visiting the sick and being a deaconess. Her family and church family made sure she attended important social functions, especially if they were in the evening or in unfamiliar neighborhoods.

Social activities should be based on the loved one's past and current interests. Most local communities offer plenty of opportunities—festivals, flower shows, musical events—that can be found in the weekend section of the newspaper.

Some of our outings included:

- Dinner at our house
- Dinner at a restaurant (select a table near few distractions)
- Church worship service, Bible study, social, or concert
- Minor league baseball game—she loved the atmosphere
- Senior community center activities
- Boat ride on the Christina River
- View Christmas decorations at the mall
- Drive to see the spring foliage, fall foliage, or Christmas lights
- Skating club show
- Tourist activities
- Concerts
- Stopping for ice cream after a medical appointment
- Visits from out-of-town family members and friends

Arriving on time or remaining until the end of an event is not necessary. To gauge how long we stayed, I observed my mother's comfort level or asked her directly if she was enjoying herself. I stopped taking her to events for which I was obligated to stay for the duration unless Alvin could take her home when she needed to leave. Some other things to consider when selecting social events are:

- Availability of handicap parking
- The proximity of parking to the event
- Amount of walking required and walking surface (carpet, tile, dirt, gravel, sand)
- Include other family members or friends?
- Can others take the loved one to this social activity and give the caregiver a break?

Holidays are an ideal time to take advantage of social outings, including family events, church concerts, fireworks, and parades. I tried to make holidays special by cooking a big meal and eating on the "good" china in the dining room. I often prepared something that was not normally served at her facility. Her facility celebrated most holidays with a special meal at noon and festivities throughout the day. Alvin picked up our mother at 4 p.m. to have a holiday celebration centered on the evening meal. As the disease progressed, a lunchtime holiday celebration worked better. Eventually, we stopped taking her out for meals because of her need to remain in a familiar environment.

Sometimes my mother would not want to leave memory care because her need for control (esteem) took priority. For instance, she refused to come to my house for a July 4th celebration because "No one told me I was going to dinner."

To: Ron, Mike   Date: 7/4/09
From: Carol   Subject: Happy 4th

Mom is being difficult today. I invited her over yesterday and told her I'd call to remind her today. She wouldn't get on the phone and said if I wanted to talk to her I needed to go there and talk to her and she wasn't going anywhere. If you talk to her before 2 p.m., mention I'm picking her up at 4:30 p.m. I'll call her at 2 p.m., and if she still says no, I won't press it.

So I began to prepare easier meals for Mom in case she did not join us and I did not expect her to stay long.

Getting my mother to participate in social activities in memory care was sometimes difficult. If I asked my mother if she was interested in an activity, she may have said no, but once she could see what was happening she may have participated.

When my mother first moved to Delaware, I tried to do something special with her every few months, but she eventually lost interest in leaving the facility, even for family gatherings. Her memory care facility met her needs for social interaction. She introduced me to the other residents (not by their name). Once another resident's family member told me, "Your mom and my mom are friends." Often, just Mom sitting with the other residents in the living room offered great socialization even though I may not have understood what they discussed. She interacted with the staff, family members of other residents, and volunteers, as well as participated in a variety of activities. She actually enjoyed being with the other residents and staff.

To: Carol, Judy, Moriah   Date: 10/19/13
From: Mike   Subject: Grandma Boyd
                                 Went Out to Lunch
There is an "Activity—Lunch Outing" on the monthly bill for
$5.64 for lunch on September 19, 2013. It is good to see they
continue to include Mom in these outings and she has the health to
participate. It can always be easier to not include her because it is
extra work, but she was included.

Initially I included spiritual needs in the social need section because
I believed spiritual needs aligned with the definition. My mother was
a devout Christian and had a great memory of biblical Scripture and
hymns. As I observed her throughout this journey, it was evident her
religious beliefs were not a need, but rather an intrinsic part of her being.
So I included opportunities to practice spirituality under the social need.
When Mom moved to Delaware, I took her to church regularly. Then
it became more difficult to have her ready early on Sunday mornings.
Instead I took her to church socials and special events and had religious
programming on the radio and television. Mom subscribed to the large
print version of *Daily Word*, a magazine of inspiration, Scripture, and
prayer. One volunteer, as part of her ministry, faithfully visited my
mother's facility and played church hymns. Mom eagerly participated
and sang hymns until she passed away.

To: Ron, Mike   Date: 3/27/09
From: Carol   Subject: Thursday
Went over to Mom's on Thursday. The choir from my former church was there so I took Mom to the lobby. She really enjoyed it. There were three other residents from Mom's area, and the caregivers took Mom back to her room afterward.

Mom participated in activities sponsored by her memory care facility including a trip to a Christian theatre with live animals and restaurants near and far. Our family events supplemented these outings. Our family appreciated the quality time spent with our mother. It was easy to see she enjoyed the events even though she may not remember them. But I will forever cherish those times.

Meeting the social need of your loved one provides a fun, different, and enriching experience. Select an event they have enjoyed in the past and engage other family members. On one of our family outings to the minor league baseball park, the team mascot greeted us as we entered the elevator. Mom's reaction was priceless. She was so surprised and laughed uncontrollably. I enjoyed watching Mom have fun. Social activities can make the caregiving journey more rewarding.

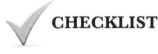 **CHECKLIST**

_____ Regularly set aside time for fun and enriching activities.
_____ Provide opportunities for your loved one to interact with family and friends.

Chapter 8

Esteem Need

• • • •

*In August 1995, long before our mother was diagnosed with
Alzheimer's, Mike, Judy, and I took her on a trip to tour New
York City. We took care of all of Mom's expenses. On the second
day in the subway station she said, "At least let me pay for
everyone's subway ticket." We were trying to treat our mother, but
she was losing her esteem. She wanted to contribute to the great
time we were having so we let her purchase our subway tickets.*

The fourth need in the pyramid is esteem and is defined as a
"desire for a high evaluation of themselves for self-respect
or self-esteem, and for the esteem of others." It includes a
desire for achievement, independence, status, dignity, or appreciation.
Satisfaction of this need leads to feelings of self-confidence and worth.
If the esteem need is not met, the person will have feelings of inferiority
and helplessness.[1]

Mom knew her memory was fading, but she never approached us
with the issue. Instead she creatively masked the problem and found
ways to cope. She wrote notes in a notebook and purchased multiple
garage door openers so she could always find one. She never posted the
laminated reminder list we provided.

To: Ron, Mike   Date: 12/28/04
From: Carol   Subject: Memory
Mom is getting slick at hiding the memory problem. When I called to tell her I probably couldn't make it, she asked, "So what's up with you?" as in, "I don't remember what is supposed to happen so I'll let you tell me."

Understanding Mom's need for esteem helped me to understand why she was opposed to having a nurse fill her pillbox when she started taking Aricept. My brothers and I placed much of our hopes in Aricept, and when the doctor finally prescribed it we wanted to ensure success. We developed what we thought was a well-thought-out plan, including a nurse to fill her pillbox and monitor for side effects.

To: Carol, Ron   Date: 4/14/04
From: Mike   Subject: "Slap in the Face"
Mom called about 9:45 p.m. to say it is a "slap in the face" to have the nurse come to fill her pillbox. She said she can do this herself and when she can no longer do this she will let us know. She said it was a waste of her time and money. I tried to argue she could get in a situation where she can't tell us and we are not there to see if this is being done correctly. I told her taking all of her medicines as prescribed is important for her health and to remain in her home.
She caught me at a wrong time because I was hungry and tired so I was pretty short with her. After some arguing I said good night.

See if you can get her to change her mind. I can't make her use the nurse.

Our plan was a severe blow to Mom's self-esteem. She had no say in the matter, and she knew she was paying for the nurse. My brothers and I focused on a successful start of Aricept and did not consider how our plan would impact her. We spent much time and anguish dealing with this situation to ensure that the nurse and medication continued.

Understanding Maslow's Hierarchy of Needs could have helped us understand our mother's need for esteem. My brothers and I could have provided more information and reinforcement about the importance of the drug. We could have said the doctor was prescribing the drug and the nurse. We could have said the nurse was only needed for the first month to verify she was taking the medication regularly. The bottom line was, we were going to do whatever necessary to ensure Mom was taking the medication, but we should have anticipated her feelings.

If someone asked Mom a question, she concocted a plausible answer if she did not know the correct response as in her response below:

To: Carol, Mike   Date: 4/15/07
From: Ron   Subject: No Subject

I talked to Mom tonight. Her voice was clear, and she sounded good for 9:30 p.m. She said she's feeling much better and thankful for good health. I mentioned her neighbor (suite mate) wasn't doing well when I was there and asked how she was doing. Mom said she didn't know. She said she (Mom) had been away. I just let that go (smiles).

Mom worked as a domestic for the first twenty-five years of her adult life. She often believed she worked at her memory care facility. Sometimes while I was visiting, she got up to remove food from the freezer for dinner. When she commented about working, I would say, "You worked hard most of your life. Now it is time to enjoy retirement." She once replied emphatically, "I do work." She firmly believed the Bible verse, "If a man will not work, he shall not eat" (2 Thessalonians 3:10). Mom believed she worked, which built her esteem and, in her mind, paid the rent. So I stopped correcting her if she mentioned working.

Throughout her life Mom was always willing to help out wherever she was needed. Memory care provided her an opportunity to help. She folded laundry and took ownership of the kitchen, which included setting the table for meals. One employee thought Mom was an employee when she first met her. Contributing to her living area was a boost to her esteem.

A phrase commonly used by the elderly is they "don't want to be a burden" to anyone. They want to be self-sufficient. Caregivers must give support without the person feeling they are a burden or helpless. If my mother was concerned about my spending money on her, sometimes I told her the item was on sale or the item was given to me. If she was concerned about my visiting her, especially if it was after dark, I told her I was in the neighborhood. Mom was not a burden to me, and I did not want her to feel that way.

Caregivers can easily help meet the need for esteem for a person in the way they interact and care for him or her. Here are some suggestions for meeting the esteem need:

- Always treat the person with dignity and respect.
- Give the person roles of dignity, allowed to go first or saying the blessing at meals.

- Celebrate his or her birthday. I bought a large cake, balloons, and gifts to celebrate with the residents and staff.
- Continue to let the loved one sign (if they can) medical forms, etc.
- Give the person opportunities to contribute. Allow the person to help with household chores, such as separating clothes for the laundry, folding clothes, setting the table, or buttering the bread.
- Compliment the loved one on what they are wearing. "That outfit matches well." "That color looks good on you."
- Provide nice, properly fitting clothing appropriate for the situation.
- Compliment the person on what they are doing. "You sure are enjoying the music."
- Compliment the loved one on his or her past abilities and accomplishments. "That blouse matches your suit well. You always had an eye for color."
- Affirm his or her statements. "Yes, it is a beautiful evening."
- Maintain grooming (hair, nails, shaving, etc.) of the person.
- Hugs, kisses, and touch are so important. Offer them liberally.
- Let the loved one make some decisions. "Do you want dinner at 4 p.m. or 5 p.m.?" "Do you want to sit on the patio?"
- Ask his or her opinion on different subjects.
- Reminisce about the person's accomplishments in the past. Only discuss accomplishments you think they remember. "You made the best homemade rolls."
- Avoid asking questions they will not remember the answer to, such as "What did you have for dinner?" or "Do you remember…?"
- Never tell others of the disease in his or her presence.

- Buy the loved one something they really like. Ron periodically sent our mother a box of candy "turtles."
- Ask relatives and friends to send the loved one cards and pictures in the mail.

Some people are natural at building esteem in others. In 2010 I took my mother to our church's Mother's Day brunch. I took her to celebrate Mother's Day and to take advantage of the spiritual and social environment. Everyone was excited to see her because she had not been to church recently. Our pastor's wife came over and greeted her warmly. She said, "Carol, where have you been hiding your mother?" An assistant minister came over and said, "Mother, it's great to see you. You really look good." And she did. (The caregiver even put make-up on my mother.) A missionary rushed out as we were leaving and told Mom, "I can't let you leave without getting a hug from you." I took my mother to the Mother's Day Brunch to meet her social need and to be in a spiritual environment. We both left the brunch with a boost to our esteem.

 CHECKLIST

_____ Tailor the list of ways to meet the esteem need for your loved one.

_____ Review some of your regular routines, phrases, or comments involving your loved one and determine if these items reduce or increase his or her esteem.

Chapter 9

Self-Actualization Need

• • • •

My mother fulfilled her need for self-actualization throughout her life. She was never afraid to push herself and learn something new. In her early forties she learned to drive, and in her late forties she enrolled in community college. Mom always had a "can do" attitude before Alzheimer's disease.

The highest need in the pyramid is self-actualization defined as man's desire for self-fulfillment or accomplishing what a person is capable of becoming. A person only has a need for self-actualization when the physiological, safety, social, and esteem needs are met.[1]

A person with or without Alzheimer's may not have a need for self-actualization even if all of his or her other needs are met, or if they do, this need is less important. A person with Alzheimer's may have met his or her need for self-fulfillment from work, volunteer activities, or raising a family. The self-actualization need is individual so tailor the activity to his or her ability. Here are suggestions to help fulfill the self-actualization need:

- Allow the person to do everything they can (as long as it is safe).

- Try new activities in which the person can be successful.
- Provide opportunities for new experiences. For instance, drive a different path.
- Follow his or her ideas or suggestions (as long as they are safe).
- Do not make the person feel helpless.

Caregivers should try some of these suggestions to test if their loved one has a strong need for self-actualization. These suggestions can be adjusted as the person declines from the disease.

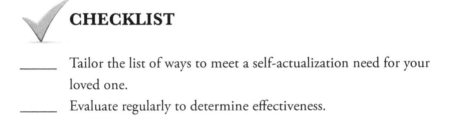 **CHECKLIST**

_____ Tailor the list of ways to meet a self-actualization need for your loved one.

_____ Evaluate regularly to determine effectiveness.

Part III

The Caregiving Principle™: Needs Filled by the Person with Alzheimer's Disease

Chapter 10

Cognitive Capability

• • • •

One day while sitting in the doctor's office, I showed my mother a Sudoku puzzle. I explained the rules, and she told me the correct number to write in the square; but she did not want to continue. I searched for ways and techniques to engage her in appropriate mind-stimulating activities. Often the issue was not could she do it, but would she do it.

The Caregiving Principle™, introduced in chapter 4, states: **Needs of the Person – Needs Filled by the Person = Needs to Be Filled by the Caregiver(s).** The "Needs Filled by the Person" with Alzheimer's disease is based on his or her cognitive capability and physical ability. The cognitive capability of a person with Alzheimer's depends on his or her cognitive capability before the disease and the amount of decline from the disease. The decline due to the illness is assessed using a scale. The Alzheimer's Association uses a three-stage scale. The Global Deterioration Scale (GDS) scale developed by Dr. Barry Reisberg (appendix 1) has seven stages.[1] My brothers and I primarily used the seven-stage scale to be aware of signs of deterioration as our mother's illness progressed. These stages are not exact and may manifest differently in different people.

Appendix 1 should not be used to conduct an assessment without a thorough medical evaluation of your loved one.

It is difficult to obtain a definitive diagnosis of Alzheimer's, so many tests rule out other causes. An exhaustive medical evaluation (chapter 3, A Watchful Eye) is critical to find out if the many reversible illnesses are causing the symptoms. Currently there is no cure for the disease, but testing will determine if Alzheimer's medication is warranted. The medication slows the progression of the disease and may lessen symptoms, such as confusion, memory loss, and problems with reasoning.

Two classes of medication are available. Cholinesterase inhibitors are prescribed during the early phase of the disease. Examples are Aricept, Exelon, and Razadyne. They slow down the process that breaks down a chemical in the brain that is believed to impact memory and thinking. The second kind of medication is N-methyl-D-aspartate (NMDA) receptor antagonist, or Namenda, and is prescribed during the later stages of the disease. It regulates the activity of an important neurotransmitter in the brain used for learning and memory.[2] Some doctors simultaneously prescribe both kinds of Alzheimer's medication.

The ability of persons with Alzheimer's disease to take care of themselves can be hindered by behaviors. Alzheimer's is a progressive illness, and the behaviors that are observed are:

- Aggression
- Agitation
- Confusion
- Depression
- Hallucinations
- Suspicion
- Sleep issues and sundowning
- Repetition
- Wandering[3]

Our mother exhibited most of the Alzheimer's behaviors in the early stages of her disease. Assisting Mom from a distance, it became impossible to distinguish between actual accounts and what my brothers and I began to call "dreams" (delusions or hallucinations). Events of her life became rearranged in her mind. It was disheartening to see our mother so distressed from the confusion, mistrust, and poor short-term memory. It was also hurtful when the mistrust was directed at those who loved her. Our constant reassurance, however, was not reassuring to her.

To: Ron, Carol   Date: 9/20/03
From: Mike   Subject: Patience

The key word needed for your stay at Mom's is PATIENCE. Keep this in mind when Mom asks you the same question over and over. Be PATIENT when Mom wants to do it her way when there is a better way. Be PATIENT when Mom wants you up and out of bed to do something you could have done later. Be PATIENT when.... It is just not worth it to exhibit frustration and anger. Mom is almost eighty-four years old, and there are things we have to just bite our tongues on and honor her desires and requests.

The above are my words meant to be helpful. I encourage myself to follow them based on my experiences this year. I directed these to you because it will be a new experience for you.

To: Ron, Mike   Date: 10/8/03
From: Carol   Subject: Break

I've been taking a break from the Mom issues but will resume this week.

I think Mom's doctor's appointment is important because they can learn what we observe. There is one question regarding behavior... and I don't mean the stubbornness. Stubbornness is just stubbornness and is part of her fight to maintain her independence. What I have seen is a tendency for her to assume the worst if something is not done when or how she expected or recollected. Example:

- I always put the lawnmower in for service, but Mike wouldn't let (doesn't want) me do it (negative tone).
- Carol didn't send whatever so something is wrong with Carol.
- Ron didn't tell me when he was coming so he's not coming, doesn't want to come, or is having problems.
- The painter wanted me to pay for the gutter guards separately so he must be a crook.

I don't know if this behavior is a symptom or not because Mom usually has a very positive outlook on things. It could be just a symptom of her being bombarded or overwhelmed with everything that is going on.

To: Carol, Mike   Date: 10/8/03

From: Ron   Subject: No Subject

As I researched loss of memory, suspicion of others is an early sign of Alzheimer's. So, Carol, I would agree with your assessment. Look over the material I'm sending. You will find it interesting.

I spoke with a couple of doctors on a geriatric ward at a psychiatric hospital regarding Aricept. They indicated the side effects of Aricept vary from person to person, but the general conclusion I got from each of them is the medication is safe, and generally speaking the side effects are minimal.

The Alzheimer's behaviors continued even after Mom began taking Aricept. My brothers and I had hoped the medication would reduce her confusion and negative behaviors, such as suspicion and hallucinations.

To: Ron, Mike   Date: 6/2/04
From: Carol   Subject: Re: (No Subject)

I said Mom was getting better, but...when I called on Sunday she thought I was in town. She thought I dropped her off at home after church and went out. Mom went to sleep, and when I wasn't there when she woke up she turned the outside light on for me. These dreams of hers are very powerful.

As usual, we'll just keep a watchful eye on her.

To: Ron, Mike   Date: 1/19/06
From: Carol   Subject: Update

I spoke with the caregiver. They do not know why we are seeing the aggressive behavior, but it could be Mom is just frustrated being around residents that are not as alert, or she realizes that is what her condition leads to.

The caregivers have seen improvement with people taking anti-anxiety medication.

I haven't had a chance to research.

Upon moving our mother to Delaware, our focus was Alzheimer's disease care. Mom's primary care physician identified a Philadelphia hospital that became an excellent resource. I prepared a packet of information for the first visit that included our mother's medical history, our concerns, and brain scans. The doctor reviewed the information before proceeding with a thorough exam. As a result, he added another Alzheimer's medication, Namenda, to her treatment plan.

The Caregiving Principle™ reminds us that the more care the person with Alzheimer's provides for himself or herself, the less care a caregiver has to provide. The difficult task is keeping the person focused despite the behaviors. Behaviors such as mistrust and suspicion are often directed at caregivers, but caregivers should not take these comments or attacks personally. It is critical to find a way to connect with the person to maximize the capability of the person.

I focused on three areas to help my mother maximize her capability. I developed these three areas based on reading, attending conferences and workshops, speaking with doctors, observing professional caregivers, and analyzing my personal interactions with my mother. These areas are linked to Maslow's Hierarchy of Needs. They are:

1. Maintain routine.
2. Minimize anxiety.
3. Engage in stimulating activity.

Maintain a Routine

My brothers and I consulted with my mother's doctor during her difficult transition to assisted living. He introduced the concept of routine because routine gives a sense of comfort and familiarity and helps meet a person's need for a sense of security. The mealtimes became the foundation of the routine with facility activities added between meals. One of the routines Mom established was meeting other residents in the parlor after breakfast.

In memory care my mother established a similar routine that my brothers and I tried to maintain. When we took her to medical appointments, we usually left after lunch and returned before dinner. If I arrived while she was eating a meal, I used that time to tidy her room so she could continue her meal uninterrupted. When I took Mom out for a meal, I maintained a time close to her 5 p.m. dinner hour. I believe she found comfort in a routine.

When my mother was admitted to the hospital, the change in routine and location was extremely disruptive. After returning home, however, Mom sometimes forgot some of her unproductive routines, such as staying up late and writing notes to the staff to reserve her room.

Minimize Anxiety

Minimizing anxiety helps the person's need for a sense of security and allows him or her to focus on the task at hand. Several techniques are used to defuse anxiety in persons with Alzheimer's.

When my mother became confused and believed something was true when it was not, my natural instinct was to correct her. Caregivers are advised to "live in the patient's world,"[4] which means not correcting or possibly lying to him or her. Agreement and "therapeutic" or "white" lies can minimize anxiety and avoid negative feelings. Often I had a difficult time following this advice. I struggled with lying to my mother, but, more important, I was concerned with my mother's next steps if I agreed with her. For instance, if my mother said, "We are leaving here tomorrow," and I agreed, her next step, if she remembered, would be to start packing her clothes. The belief is that the person will forget the next step, but they did not know my mom. The caregivers would make a comment to Mom to "live in the patient's world." Sometimes she would remember, and the next step was a telephone call to me: "Carol, they told me you took my car."

I had to rethink how I handled "living in the patient's world." My focus was to reduce the anxiety in both of us. I asked myself, does it matter if what Mom believes is not true? If her belief did not cause more anxiety, I just let it go, most times. But if she was concerned about where she lived or concerned about her rent being paid, I corrected her or said or did whatever was necessary to eliminate those negative thoughts.

Redirection of a person with Alzheimer's is another technique to reduce anxiety. Sometimes just changing the subject is adequate. "Look at the red bird flying over there." The hope is that the person will forget what happened before the comment about the red bird. When my mother looked like she may say something negative, I said something positive to set the tone. Another method is what I call the name-drop technique. In general, I believe my mother's generation was more agreeable to ideas, thoughts, or opinions from men. I tried to take advantage of her view and use the name-drop method. "Mike thinks it is best if...." The staff used the name-drop technique and said, "Carol wants you to...." One time Mom replied, "I am the mother, and Carol is the daughter. She does not tell me what to do." These techniques can be extremely useful, and most worked, but not all of the time.

To: Carol, Mike   Date: 7/13/07
From: Ron   Subject: Re: Mom

Mom's illness is so baffling. Something that may bother her yesterday, she's fine with today. Then she can be so alert and on most points and later lost, very forgetful, and constantly repetitive in speech. I smile at some of our techniques used to assist her when she is not focused. Mom is something else.

Music has been proven as an effective tool to improve the mood of persons with Alzheimer's. Caregivers have used personalized playlists for waking, bathing, dressing, or any activity, including waiting in a doctor's office.[5] Music can boost the cognitive skills possibly through a process of resynchronization as the music rhythm stimulates timing and processes in the brain.[6]

At some point, the anxiety associated with Alzheimer's disease may warrant more medication. My brothers and I had no desire to place our mother on anti-anxiety or anti-psychotic drugs. But she regularly was overly worried about something. "How long can I stay here?" "How much does it cost?" I began to feel anxious just sitting next to her. Mom needed medication in addition to the daily Aricept and Namenda to take the edge off.

To: Ron, Mike   Date: 6/4/07
From: Carol   Subject: Incident
Mom had a bad night last night. The caregiver called at 12:30 a.m. saying Mom was up and aggressive with the caregivers. I believe she thought she was at her home in Cleveland and there were people in her house. She threatened to call the police. She wouldn't go to bed until they left.

So Alvin and I went over, and she went to bed. We remained for a while, but she didn't get up. They said she's fine this morning. I hope this is just a one-time thing.

In July 2007, my brothers and I agreed that anti-anxiety medication was warranted. I was hopeful approaching the neurologist because we had discussed his medication philosophy during our mother's first visit. He understood our reluctance, and we were especially concerned about the side effects of anti-psychotic drugs.[7] The doctor had mentioned that if medication was warranted he would tailor the selected drug and the dosage for the specific situation. I appreciated his one-size-does-not-fit-all approach and his knowledge of the options. We discussed Mom's behaviors, and he prescribed an extremely low dose of an anti-anxiety medication with a plan to increase if needed. We saw a remarkable improvement in her behavior with the initial dosage. It was much easier having a conversation, and she was less concerned about her ability to continue to live there. Mom no longer exhibited the anxious look or the nervous tapping of her foot. We were pleased that such a low dose made a significant improvement in her well-being...another ray of hope.

To: Ron, Mike   Date: 7/11/07
From: Carol   Subject: Anxiety
I spoke with the caregiver. She sees an improvement in Mom since she started taking the anti-anxiety medication. She said they had no problem getting her on the bus to go to lunch today. Unfortunately I missed seeing her while I was there, but I prefer she get out.

Engage in Stimulating Activity

Stimulating activity may slow the mental decline and help a person reach his or her full potential (self-actualization). It was difficult finding stimulating things my mother could and would do on her own. She had enjoyed word search puzzles but now would not open the puzzle book unless prompted. My mother read the newspaper regularly during the early phases of the disease, and I knew she had some level of comprehension.

Puzzles and games are mind stimulating and fun. Some suggestions are Bingo, UNO, Wheel of Fortune, Dominoes, and card games. Participation is important. Make the game fun even if the rules are not followed. Multiple books and articles on activities are offered for persons with Alzheimer's disease.

Almost any project or activity the person with Alzheimer's disease engages in can stimulate the mind. On a doctor's visit my mother helped me find the correct address, the suite number from the building directory, and the elevator. On another visit I read a magazine article with Mom, and we discussed it while waiting in the examining room.

To: Ron, Mike   Date: 11/15/07
From: Carol   Subject: Update

I stopped by Mom's today. She had on a different outfit, and she was doing well. I may take her to the Sunday Breakfast Mission on Saturday when the youth ministry goes to sort food for Thanksgiving baskets.

Alzheimer's behaviors can prevent a person from meeting his or her need even if he or she is capable of doing so. Maintaining a routine, reducing anxiety, medication, and providing stimulating activity helped my mother maximize her capability.

✓ CHECKLIST

_____ Document Alzheimer's behaviors and obtain a proper medical diagnosis and treatment plan for your loved one.

_____ Establish a daily routine.

_____ Reduce anxiety by using techniques such as "living in the patient's world," redirection (changing the subject), and name-dropping.

_____ Develop a playlist of songs from your loved one's music collection.

_____ Identify one or two stimulating activities your loved one enjoys.

Chapter 11

Physical Ability

• • • •

My father died in 1987 from cancer. Sometimes I wondered if a physical ailment was easier to manage than Alzheimer's disease. Physical ailments are easier to understand but bring their share of pain and sickness. In reality, persons with Alzheimer's also have physical ailments. Managing both is overwhelming.

The "Needs Filled by the Person" portion of The Caregiving Principle™ is also based on the physical ability. Normal physical changes in an aging body include slower reflexes, arthritic joints, loss of peripheral vision, and decreased mobility.[1] At the 2009 Delaware Alzheimer's Education Conference, the facilitators simulated what it is like to have Alzheimer's. The simulation took into account many of the physical changes of an aging body. Popcorn kernels were placed in our shoes; we wore earplugs and vision-altering eyeglasses; some of our fingers were wrapped to reduce dexterity. Then we performed basic tasks such as folding laundry, finding a name in a telephone book, and telephone dialing. This simulation helped me to understand what my mother was experiencing as her body aged and declined from Alzheimer's.

Persons with Alzheimer's disease are often elderly and may experience pain from arthritis, past injuries, or a new injury and illness. As the disease progresses, they may not be able to effectively communicate pain so caregivers need to pay close attention to facial expressions, utterances, and behaviors.

Ninety-five percent of my mother's medical appointments were related to maintaining her physical health. She received most of the recommended adult vaccinations such as tetanus, influenza, and pneumococcal (pneumonia). Mom showed signs of chronic lung disease. Yet she was blessed with good physical health well into her early nineties.

A knee replacement was the first surgery Mom had after my brothers and I assumed responsibility for her care. We decided the surgery would enhance her quality of life, but we were concerned about the effects of the anesthesia. We did our research and spoke to the doctors. The consensus was the anesthesia may make her "goofy" for a few days, but she should return to her pre-surgery mental state.

The bigger issue with Alzheimer's disease patients and hospital visits is they may not remember they are in a hospital or why.

To: Ron, Mike   Date: 5/17/05
From: Carol   Subject: Tuesday, May 17th update

When I returned to the hospital last night, Mom was against the side of the bed. She said she had gone to the bathroom, but the nurses don't believe she did. It was a major accident about to happen. She had unplugged the leg circulators, oxygen, catheter, and the blood drain from her knee. It is a blessing we didn't find her on the floor.

She is somewhat disoriented, but I don't believe it is any worse than normal. She woke up a couple of times in the night and asked what time we had to be at the hospital not realizing she was at the hospital. She is not taking as much pain medication as she could. They started her back on her normal meds.

This simple, planned hospital stay for knee replacement surgery became a challenge for us. I knew if our mother got out of bed again she could have worse consequences so I spent the night with her. I was prepared to stay the second night when the hospital offered a sitter, someone to watch and help Mom. I was extremely grateful for this help, a ray of hope.

Many hospitals have sitters, and I began to alert the staff of our mother's situation upon admittance. In one instance, the hospital assigned another patient to her room who also needed a sitter. Some families will hire a private caregiver to stay with a loved one when he or she enters a hospital or a rehabilitation center.

The first year our mother was in Delaware, my brothers and I focused on Alzheimer's care and pressing medical care. The second year we focused on less urgent care such as eye, dental, and feet because providing medical care to the entire body helped her quality of life. The probability of contracting some illnesses diminishes with age, so discuss with your loved one's doctor the preventive tests based on age and family history. My brothers and I evaluated the potential benefits and negative impact before having Mom endure any procedure or surgery. For instance, we believed the improved visual clarity from cataract surgery might have eliminated some confusion.

My mother had a cataract surgically removed from her left eye in 2008 and another removed from her right eye in 2010. Sometimes the doctor removes the lens from the eyeglasses of the eye that had the surgery. I knew this practice would cause Mom to think her glasses were broken so we placed a clear lens in my mother's glasses until the eye healed and the correct lens was prescribed. The clear lens allowed her to see correctly out of one eye and not be concerned.

Hospitalizations were extremely unsettling for my mother. First of all, she did not always recognize where she was. I learned to remove Mom's clothes when she was admitted to prevent her from trying to leave. Even if my mother only got dressed, it could cause a disruption in her care. Hospitalizations were also unsettling because of the testing, monitoring, treatment, and questions from the doctors and staff. I worked with her doctor to keep abreast of the diagnostic test results and treatment plan. I worked with the hospital staff to ensure the doctor's plan was being followed and to check on Mom's well-being. I constantly reassured and re-oriented Mom to ensure she was doing her part (eating, physical therapy, etc.) to get released. A higher dose of anti-anxiety medication was prescribed during hospitalizations. At the recommendation of her doctor, I purchased a small stuffed animal. Eventually, the pink bunny became a familiar item she could have at home, in the hospital, and in the rehabilitation facility.

Some hospitalizations may require rehabilitation afterward. The rehabilitation facility is another unfamiliar place that may cause confusion.

Physical activity is recommended for good health, but Mom never participated regularly in the daily exercises offered by either of her facilities. She walked frequently from her room to the common areas. For trips outside I let Mom walk to and from my car in the parking lot unless she was physically unable or in inclement weather. I also encouraged her to walk with me on the patio.

Providing preventive medical care keeps the loved one from suffering unnecessarily. Caregivers must evaluate the benefit and risk of medical procedures. Consult with a doctor to determine what screenings are appropriate based on age and family history. Regular medical care can improve the quality of life of a loved one.

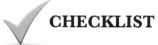 **CHECKLIST**

_____ Keep current on medical screenings and appointments. Ensure your loved one is taking his or her medications.

_____ Select a hospital to manage the care of your loved one because all services are in the same location (maybe a different wing or building) and the doctors can coordinate care. Select highly recommended doctors who interact well with persons with Alzheimer's.

_____ Prepare a contingency plan for an emergency room visit and/or hospitalization.

Part IV

Tools for the Caregiver to Fulfill Needs

Chapter 12

Faith

• • • •

I had to step out on faith when my brothers and I decided to move our mother to Delaware. I believed the move was right, but would the move kill Mom's spirit or her will to live? We selected a facility based on its ability to meet Mom's short- and long-term needs. But something was telling me it was not the right place. I continued to search, and God led us to a facility that was not on our initial list. Although my mother's transition was difficult, I am convinced we made the right decision to move Mom to the newly found memory care facility in Delaware.

My mother was my living example of what faith in God can do. She was a deaconess in her church, and my parents were extremely dedicated to the National Baptist Deacons Convention, Inc. As Mom lost her memory, she never lost her faith. Mom's strong faith encouraged me throughout this journey when I visited her. She was a constant reminder of the meaning of faith and the power of God.

*"Now faith is the substance of things hoped for, the evidence of
things not seen."*
(Hebrews 11:1)

My faith in God teaches that I will have trials and these trials will
make me strong.

*"Therefore I take pleasure in infirmities, in reproaches, in
necessities, in persecutions, in distresses for Christ's sake: for when
I am weak, then am I strong."*
(2 Corinthians 12:10)

and

*"And we know that all things work together for good to them that
love God, to them who are the called according to his purpose."*
(Romans 8:28)

Each challenge I overcome provides strength and encouragement
for the challenge that lies ahead. My walk on this journey has helped me
embrace these verses:

*"Nay, in all these things we are more than conquerors through
him that loved us."*
(Romans 8:37)

and

"I can do all things through Christ which strengtheneth me."
(Philippians 4:13)

I attended a glorious church ceremony that elevated some of our senior deacons to emeritus deacon. These deacons, who are trained and prepared to pray with our members, had faithfully served for multiple decades. Each deacon was introduced with his favorite Scripture when confronting persons who were experiencing illness or death of a loved one. They had multiple Scriptures for different life situations.

As a caregiver, I had to be trained and prepared to handle a wide range of situations. Sometimes I found myself with feelings of frustration, guilt, fear, and mental fatigue. I found my state of mind could directly impact Mom's state of mind or her behavior so I had to manage my emotions. In the midst of a situation I needed the right words to comfort myself. I did not always have the ability to reach for a Bible, so I relied on the words or songs that were playing on the gospel radio station in my car. Many times I heard the right Scripture or song for the situation. Then I became more proactive. I learned, like the deacons, having prayer and the right Scripture or song at my fingertips is a powerful tool. The prayer called on God, and the Scripture or song helped to manage my emotions in a positive and encouraging way. For example, when I was extremely frustrated with my mother or her situation, I meditated on:

"I will lift up mine eyes unto the hills, from whence cometh my help.
My help cometh from the Lord, which made heaven and earth."
(Psalm 121:1-2)

Or I may have sung or hum the hymn,

What a friend we have in Jesus,
All our sins and griefs to bear!
What a privilege to carry
Everything to God in prayer.
Oh, what peace we often forfeit,

Oh, what needless pain we bear,
All because we do not carry
Everything to God in prayer.[1]
Lyrics by Joseph M. Scriven

The behavior I struggled with the most was patience. Persons with Alzheimer's disease ask the same questions over and over and over again, and they also have impaired reasoning. I had to look to Romans:

"By whom also we have access by faith into this grace wherein
we stand, and rejoice in hope of the glory of God.
And not only so, but we glory in tribulations also: knowing that
tribulation worketh patience;
And patience, experience; and experience, hope:"
(Romans 5:2-4)

My patience has grown tremendously, but I continually work on it. A song I sang to encourage my patience was "He Looked beyond My Fault (and Saw My Need)" by Dottie Rambo:

Amazing grace shall always be my song of praise
For it was grace that bought my liberty
I do not know just why He came to love me so
He looked beyond my fault and saw my need.[2]

I was not a perfect caregiver, but God looked beyond my faults. I had to look beyond my faults, beyond my impatience, beyond Mom's illness, beyond her disruptive behaviors, and understand and meet her needs.

At times I felt everything was going wrong, and I knew I needed a complete attitude adjustment. The song that helped me was "I Smile" by Kirk Franklin. When I first heard the song, the only word I knew was "smile," and just that one word with the upbeat rhythm encouraged my soul. After hearing the song again, the lyrics that jumped out at me were:

I almost gave up, but a power that I can't explain,
Fell from heaven like a shower.[3]

Many times on this Alzheimer's journey I wanted to give up, but I could not. During these times I had to temporarily withdraw from the situation. Jesus, in the midst of healing and ministering, withdrew from the crowds and disciples and went to be alone with God for prayer and rejuvenation.[4] Like Jesus, I had to reach out to God for help. I had to reach out to receive God's amazing grace.

Physical and mental fatigue is a regular part of this journey. I tried to get my required rest and not overextend myself, but I was not always successful. A telephone call about Mom could quickly make an already hectic day more hectic. I reminded myself:

"Finally, my brethren, be strong in the Lord, and in the power of
his might."
(Ephesians 6:10)

I reached to God for strength or sometimes thought about the times Mom did things for me during my childhood when I knew she was tired.

The challenges along the Alzheimer's journey create uncertainty and sometimes fear, a looming fear of illness, rapid decline, and death. I was fearful the first time I watched Mom taken to the hospital in an ambulance with respiratory issues. The Scripture I relied on then was:

"For God hath not given us the spirit of fear; but of power, and
of love, and of a sound mind."
(2 Timothy 1:7)

I could not be afraid. I had to have a sound mind to ensure that my brothers and I were making the right decisions for our mother. So during periods of fear the song I may have sung was "Through It All."

> *I've had many tears and sorrows,*
> *I've had questions for tomorrow;*
> *There've been times I didn't know right from wrong,*
> *But in every situation God gave me blessed consolation*
> *That my trials come to only make me strong.*
>
> *Chorus*
> *Through it all,*
> *Through it all,*
> *I've learned to trust in Jesus,*
> *I've learned to trust in God.*
> *Through it all,*
> *Through it all,*
> *I've learned to depend upon His Word.*[5]
>
> Andrae Crouch

My faith in God is the source of my encouragement, support, and strength. As I prayed regularly, attended worship services, participated in church ministry, studied God's Word, and listened to Christian radio and television, God increased my faith. My faith in God was the most powerful tool along this Alzheimer's journey.

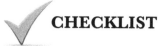 **CHECKLIST**

_____ Develop or strengthen your relationship with God by becoming an active member of a Bible-believing church, by studying the Bible, and through prayer.

_____ Prepare your list of Bible verses, quotations, and songs to have at your fingertips as you encounter negative emotions and situations.

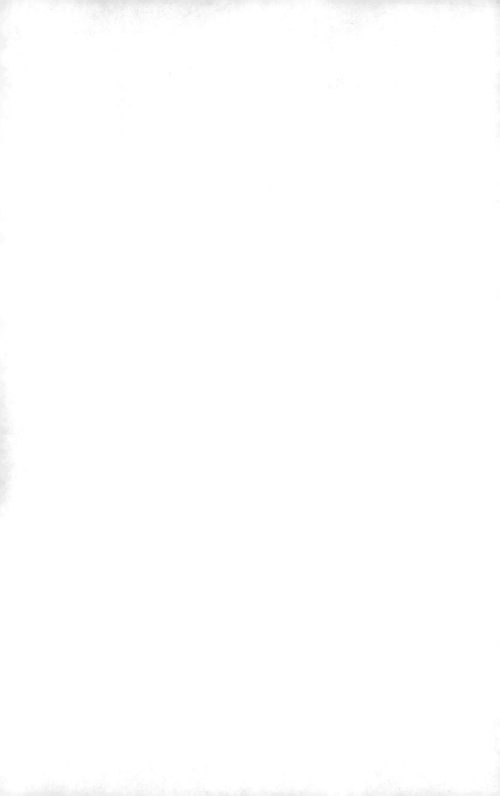

Chapter 13

Resources

• • • •

I reached out for solutions when encountering a problem. My brothers and I installed a telephone for our mother in Delaware, and her first few phone bills were exorbitant. She called anyone (directory assistance, family, airlines, etc.) who could help her return to Cleveland. The telephone company explained a feature that blocked calls we did not want Mom to make. I updated her telephone contact list to show dialing instructions from Delaware. Her phone bill quickly moved to a normal range, and Mom was able to maintain contact with her family and friends.

The best source of Alzheimer's information is the Alzheimer's Association, and it should be your first stop. Periodically I visited the local office to browse through the pamphlets and library. The staff is extremely helpful and knowledgeable. I used the list of Delaware assisted-living facilities, nursing homes, and caregiver support groups and found the lists extremely valuable. I have learned a great deal from the workshops and networking with other family and professional caregivers. The 2010 Annual Delaware Dementia Conference featured Dr. Peter Rabins, co-author of *The 36-Hour Day.* The 2017 conference discussed the stigma associated with Alzheimer's disease and how it impacts care. Even the fundraisers, such as the Walk to End Alzheimer's, are designed to educate and raise awareness about the disease. The website (www.alz.org) has an extensive virtual library of information for all aspects and stages of the illness and is updated regularly. Librarians are available by phone, email, or in a chat room to answer questions. Families can access training online. Annually the Alzheimer's Association issues a comprehensive report on the state of the disease in America called *Alzheimer's Disease Facts and Figures.* It includes statistics and information on new developments, diagnosis, prevalence, and caregivers. Many facts in this book are from the Alzheimer's Association.[1]

The Alzheimer's Association provides a number of services to support caregivers. There is the twenty-four-hour, seven-day-a-week helpline (800 272-3900),[2] Medic Alert + Safe Return (to reunite lost persons with Alzheimer's with family),[3] and Trialmatch (to identify candidates for clinical trials).[4] An Alzheimer's caregiver support group can be an extremely useful tool because of the collective knowledge of the facilitator and other caregivers. The Alzheimer's Association offers specialty support groups such as one for men, for African Americans, or for those diagnosed with early onset dementia. Caregivers not participating in a support group should speak regularly to other Alzheimer's caregivers.

The Alzheimer's Disease Education and Referral Center (ADEAR) is a service of the National Institute on Aging (NIA). The center has a wealth of information including Alzheimer's research, news, and information for caregivers.[5] AARP.org also has useful information on caregiving.

The Alzheimer's Store has products useful for caregivers and persons with Alzheimer's in many stages of the disease. Examples are medicine dispensers, photo dialing telephones, door and window alarms, and motion detectors.[6]

Investigate local resources offered in your city or county. Mike had a habit of looking at pamphlets and bulletin boards in doctor offices, hospitals, and government offices to identify additional local resources. My family found valuable resources from the local Office on Aging in Cleveland. They provided social workers, legal consultants, van service, Medicare counselors, Meals on Wheels, a personal emergency response system, and applications for local, state, and federal programs. In Delaware, the *Guide to Services for Older Delawareans and Persons with Disabilities* is a directory of information and resources. Look for similar resources in your area from community and nonprofit organizations that offer services for the elderly.

My employer provided access to a work-life company that aids employees who are balancing life issues with work. This company was extremely useful and helped us design the meeting (intervention) to persuade Mom to move to assisted living. They also provided a list of facilities in Ohio and Delaware and information on legal documents needed.

The Family and Medical Leave Act (FMLA) allows employees to take twelve weeks of unpaid, job-protected leave in a twelve-month period to care for an immediate family member. Family leave can be beneficial after the Alzheimer's diagnosis, during a hospitalization, or while changing your loved one's living situation. FMLA can be used intermittently during the twelve-month period to accommodate shorter times away from work such as medical appointments.[7] Caregivers should work with the human resources department to understand the details. Employers may provide other types of assistance such as working late or swapping shifts.

I developed a good library of books on Alzheimer's disease. Every book and pamphlet had useful information, a different approach, or a word of encouragement. I read the section that applied to Mom's current situation. Revisit your personal library periodically as your loved one advances to another stage of the disease.

Many resources are available to help caregivers on their journey. Reading, visiting the Alzheimer's Association website, and attending classes take time but can reduce the stress of caregiving.

✓ CHECKLIST

_____ Visit your local Alzheimer's Association office, speak with the staff, and browse the library.

_____ Create your personal Alzheimer's library with information from the Alzheimer's Association, bookstores, and other resources.

_____ Visit the Alzheimer's Association website at www.alz.org. Select one pressing issue to research.

Chapter 14

Communication

• • • •

The most important communication was between my mother and me. Sometimes I sat with her and just let her talk. Mom also called me at home. She never spoke long. She just wanted to know we were okay. Sometimes Mom called multiple times a night, not remembering she called earlier. Most times I pretended she had not called. Occasionally she called at 12:30 a.m. or 2 a.m. with a concern that had been handled. Even though I was asleep when she called, I was patient. I knew someday these calls would end.

Communication (verbal, visual, and listening) was important to understand our mother's feelings and concerns. When she lived alone, I called almost every night to remind her to take her Aricept. My brothers called her regularly. We followed up our conversations with a letter if she needed important information such as our visit dates. We encouraged her to keep important information on her bulletin board, which included a calendar.

In Delaware our mother called my brothers and me almost every night, and I visited her regularly. A church member recommended I not visit every day because of my full-time position that included travel. This was a personal decision, but the advice served me well. If we were dealing with issues or if she was in the hospital, I visited multiple times a day. We discovered it was important to keep her grounded; regular visits and contacts reassured her. Ron increased his calling frequency when I traveled. I visited Mom often even if I could not stay long. If I had a tennis match in her neighborhood, I may have visited with her before and after the match. A friend was faithfully taking her mother to visit her aunt with Alzheimer's. They were both mentally drained after the three-hour visit. My friend was so happy when I suggested shorter, more frequent visits.

Communicating (speaking and listening) with a person with Alzheimer's can be difficult. Often the questions have a deeper meaning. For instance, when I was out with Mom, she continuously asked the time. The real question was, "Will I return home by mealtime?" Mostly she only needed reassurance she had a place to return to. Purposely, I kept our conversations light and upbeat. I used humor to make her smile or laugh. I did not discuss negative news such as illness or the death of family members or friends. Mike and I did not tell her about the death of her son or two sisters. I screened her mail after the death of family members so she did not find out about the death from a sympathy card.

Even though I lived in a different city from my mother most of my adult life, I knew her quite well. I could tell when she was telling the truth or trying to mask that she did not know an answer. When Mom became less verbal during the later stages of the disease, it was amazing how well she communicated with facial expressions. I caught myself many times saying, "She gave me a look that said. . . ."

To: Mike   Date: 3/9/13
From: Carol   Subject: 3/9

I am at the hospital with Mom. Her lunch was still here so I just finished feeding her. I will come back at dinnertime to make sure she eats. Mom has that fed-up look on her face. She is ready to leave and return to her memory care facility. I reinforce that she is getting stronger every day.

Communications should consider the needs of the person. When I took Mom on outings, I communicated multiple times she would return home. I filled in gaps that may have been in her mind. For instance, I picked her up one evening after her dinner to attend a minor league baseball outing sponsored by our church. I planned to have my dinner at the stadium. At the stadium, I said, "You may not be hungry since you just had dinner, but if you want something I will get it for you. Or maybe you'll just want dessert." She then knew she had eaten and did not have to wonder why I did not purchase food for her.

In my communication with Mom, I:

- Described persons based on their relationship to her: "Your son Ron...."
- Used simpler sentences.
- Gave my mother adequate time to respond.
- Listened for deeper meanings to her questions.
- Gauged the conversation from her reaction. Sometimes mentioning someone from the past was upsetting if she could not remember the person.
- Kept conversations positive even if she had a negative attitude.
- Learned to incorporate what had happened and what was going to happen in my regular conversations to keep her informed.

- Sometimes spoke in extremes to get a reaction from her. If someone was skating on television, I might say, "Let's put some skates on you and go skating into the sunset." This started a conversation or at a minimum got a laugh.
- Felt comfortable just being with her and not saying a word.

Two great resources for improving communication with a person with Alzheimer's disease are:

- *Communication, Tips for Successful Communication during All Stages of Alzheimer's Disease*, Alzheimer's Association.[1]
- *Learning to Speak Alzheimer's: A Groundbreaking Approach for Everyone Dealing with the Disease* by Joanne Koenig Coste.[2]

As the disease progressed, our mother did not initiate much conversation, but she would let me know if she needed something. She did not always know the correct word to use, or she may have used the wrong word. My brothers and I learned not to speak as if she was not present. We noticed Mom was very much aware of what was going on. The lack of speech of persons with Alzheimer's is not an indication they cannot hear or understand. Many of us have had a thought, and the next words out of our mouths assumed we had spoken our thought. I think our mother believed she had spoken her thought.

I communicated regularly with my brothers through emails. Emails were effective because everyone stayed informed, each sibling received the same information, and we could respond at our convenience. Time differences, work schedules, or travel were not issues. We could ask questions, offer suggestions, and send information. We clarified and expanded on our ideas via email. Our emails documented our decisions, tasks, and responsibilities. Our frequent communication provided a consistent story when discussing issues with our mother.

When dealing with a major issue like a hospitalization, we may have each sent two to three emails a day. The dialog was beneficial, because often in the middle of a medical crisis, for instance, my focus was the well-being of our mother. My brothers could evaluate the situation, research the condition, make recommendations, and suggest questions for the doctor or staff. During normal times, we sent maybe one or two emails a week. Sometimes we spoke by phone or sent information by postal mail. I made mailing labels for my brothers to facilitate communication by mail with each other and with our mother. An added benefit of our frequent communication was that we were more engaged in each other's personal lives, which enriched us all and made our family stronger.

To: Carol, Mike   Date: 11/2/03
From: Ron   Subject: Re: Doctor response
I just sent you a response with my views on the issues at hand. And after reading your emails today, I see we're all on the same page. GREAT!!!!!!!!!!!!!!!!!!!!

My brothers and I also communicated in writing or by telephone with our mother's siblings because they did not regularly use email. Ron normally handled these letters and calls. The purpose was to update her siblings on her status if she approached them with concerns. For instance, Ron sent a letter to them to tell of her impending move to assisted living. Ron was a critical link to her siblings, and when he passed away we did not maintain communications with her siblings as well. We never reassigned his tasks.

Families now have many more options for communicating, such as text messages, social media, FaceTime, etc. It is important to establish guidelines on what information will be shared outside the immediate family.

I used faxes, letters, or phone calls to communicate with Mom's doctors, especially if her situation changed. For the first doctor's visit I wrote a letter summarizing our mother's history and current concerns. My brothers provided input to these letters to ensure all of our concerns were stated clearly and concisely. I attached copies of medical information and sometimes faxed to the doctor in advance. The letter method worked extremely well, and I did not have to mention issues or negative behavior in Mom's presence. We were fortunate to have had doctors who spoke directly to her. One time her doctor was giving her instructions, and she said, "You need to make sure my daughter understands that."

It was extremely important to communicate with the staff and caregivers at my mother's facility. I kept the caregivers informed of doctor recommendations, expected visitors, and planned outings. They used this information to monitor for changes in her health or behavior and to have her ready for trips or guests. The caregivers were good at initiating communication with me. They observed Mom daily and could identify when a change occurred in her behavior, eating and sleeping habits, or health.

Occasionally I attended meetings for residents and family members. I spoke and shared experiences with the family members of other residents. We were an informal support group and provided emotional support for each other. We cared for and interacted with all the residents in the area.

Each time our mother moved, I mailed decorative change-of-address cards so family and friends could maintain contact with her. Sometimes while visiting with her, I called a friend or family member. I ensured

Mom sent Christmas cards to about thirty family members and friends each year. I created address and return address labels, which helped. In 2009 I started using picture Christmas cards, which simplified the writing. Everyone enjoyed the pictures and liked seeing that Mom was doing well. She was blessed to have such great family and friends.

Family and friends should identify ways to connect and communicate with the loved one even as the illness progresses. Caregivers must maintain communications with other family members, friends, and care providers. Determine the best time and form of communication. Effective communication can make the journey less stressful and more rewarding.

 CHECKLIST

_____ Improve communication with your loved one by reading the recommended materials.

_____ Keep appropriate family members, friends, and care providers informed of your loved one's situation.

_____ Determine the best form of communication for the persons or institutions you communicate with regularly.

_____ Reassign tasks as the circle of support changes.

Chapter 15

Organization

• • • •

Providing care for someone is rewarding, but stressful. Losing a written prescription, forgetting a medical appointment, and running out of medications have caused stress in my life. Organization relieved some caregiving stress.

Assuming responsibility for a loved one's affairs is much easier with organizational tools. My brothers and I developed several tools that worked for us and can easily adapt to your situation. I have included some tools that others have used.

Memory Aid – Notebook

Mike provided our mother with a notebook to keep track of the things she needed to do. The notebook helped us understand what was going on because she kept good notes and often recorded her thoughts or concerns.

Things-to-Do List/Visit Summary

When our mother was living in Cleveland, Mike and I visited her separately on a monthly basis. The things-to-do list helped us organize our activities during our visits. My brothers and I worked to prioritize what needed to be accomplished. We always had more list than we had time, but the list served to document the needs. What was not completed on a trip we hoped would be completed on the next visit. Our activities and progress were documented in a visit summary. Two partial visit summaries/trip reports are in chapter 27, Be Grateful for God's Rays of Hope. A partial, sample things-to-do list is below:

To: Ron, Mike   Date: 10/17/03

From: Carol   Subject: 10/25-27 To-Do List

I'm getting my to-do list for my 10/25-27 visit. I still have a lot to do. Some items can be done before the visit, but I've developed an all-inclusive list based on all the emails going back and forth.

- Medical

    We need to come to agreement on what our position is for the start of Aricept. I believe we should present the data to the doctors and let them make the call. The doctors should make the decision based on:

    - Neuropsych evaluation
    - Our observations (memory, inability to deal with complex issues, behavior changes)
    - Genetic information – Ron, please get age at which our aunt started showing signs of Alzheimer's.
    - Ruling out other causes of symptoms

    If Aricept is prescribed, we will need a monitoring plan and an abort strategy.

- Issues to discuss with Mom
    - Importance of social worker visits
    - Reinforce the importance of visiting the senior center.
    - House and car key location

- Emergency response system – continue to lay groundwork
- Nutritional supplement – twice a day
- Rest
- Other Tasks
  - Review new mail/paperwork
  - Sew front door curtains
  - Find garage door key

To: Carol, Ron   Date: 10/18/03
From: Mike   Subject: Re: 10/25-27 To-Do List

I saw your master list and was immediately overwhelmed. It got worse when I realized some items were missing. You do a great job capturing the many things to do. Below are a few comments and some additions....

Lots of stuff. Don't be overwhelmed. Things will get added while you are there. Don't lose sight of the main purpose for your visit.

Filing Cabinet

Mike purchased a two-drawer filing cabinet to organize our mother's paperwork at her home. We had files for bills, doctor visits, and automobile, to name a few. We encouraged Mom to use the cabinet, but at best, she placed the paperwork on top of the cabinet.

To organize our mother's paperwork at my home, I purchased a portable plastic file case on wheels. My brothers and Alvin knew where Mom's paperwork resided, and it kept her paperwork separated from my personal papers.

Non-Monthly Bills

Mike listed our mother's non-monthly bills and the due dates. This served as a reminder and helped her manage her cash flow when she managed her finances. The list included real estate taxes and car, homeowner's, and long-term care insurance.

Online Banking

Online banking or accounting software packages can simplify the management of finances. The loved one can continue to initiate transactions, but the caregiver should have access to electronic monitoring to ensure all bills are being paid. When the loved one can no longer manage this task, the caregiver can easily assume this responsibility.

Passwords

Over time a person accumulates a large number of passwords for the ATM, financial accounts, medical accounts, shopping, insurance, and so on. Start collecting and protecting the passwords of your loved one.

Contact List

I created a laminated list of the home, work, and cell phone numbers of immediate family members, a friend, and the social worker. The laminated card was created in two sizes, a large card for the house and car and a smaller card for the wallet. These cards were given to Mom and everyone on the list and others so they could contact us if an issue arose.

Medication List

I kept a list of our mother's medications with the dosage. It is important to revise this list regularly, especially after a hospitalization. A medication list is needed for most medical visits.

Medication Tracking

Some facilities require that they supply and administer all medications and others let the family supply medications. I developed a spreadsheet to keep track of when I needed to reorder, but this became too cumbersome. Eventually I managed to synchronize the ordering of most of her prescription medication.

List of Doctors

Many assisted-living and memory care facilities have doctors who visit regularly. These doctors are usually primary care physicians, but specialists such as podiatrists or physical therapists may also visit. My brothers and I chose to use outside doctors for Mom. One of the most useful tools I developed was a spreadsheet with our mother's medical providers. It included the name, address, phone, fax, hours, and recommended frequency of visits of her medical providers (table 3). My brothers also had a copy.

Table 3

Medical Providers

PROVIDER	SPECIALTY	ADDRESS	PHONE	FAX	HOURS	Q1	Q2	Q3	Q4
Dr. Gerry Attics	PCP	1823 Primary Road			M-Th 8-5, F 8-12	X	X	X	X
Dr. Mary Childress	OB GYN	89 Pamper Place			M-Th 8-6		X	X	
Dr. Miriam Foote	Podiatrist	1 Walking Way			M-Th 8-5		X		X
Lab Testing	Laboratory	339A Positive Place			M-F 8-6, S 8-12				
Pharmacy	Local	56 Pill Blvd.			24 hours				
Pharmacy	Mail Order	PO Box 1708							
Dr. Harry Reason	Neurologist	196 Learning Lane			W-F 1-5	X		X	
Dr. Elizabeth Wind	Lungs	4417 Airway Road			M-F 8-5		X		X
Urgent Care	Urgent Care	18 Vital Blvd.			M-S 8-9, Sun 10-6				
X-Ray	X-Ray	4 Image Road			M-F 8-6, S 8-12				
Scheduled Visits/quarter						2	4	3	3

Our mother averaged ten to fifteen regularly scheduled doctor's appointments every year. The doctor list helped us to manage, schedule, and coordinate appointments proactively. I scheduled appointments during a two-day period each quarter. My brothers coordinated their Delaware visits so they could take Mom to her appointments. This allowed them to meet her doctors and helped me tremendously by reducing my responsibilities.

Doctor Visit Form

My brothers and I started using a doctor visit form that listed issues since the last visit, medical visits to specialists, questions, and prescription refills needed. The form ensured we covered everything that was needed during the visit. It was especially helpful when my brothers took her to an appointment.

Calendar

A properly used calendar is a must when managing schedules for your loved one, yourself, and possibly other family members.

To: Ron, Mike   Date: 4/5/06
From: Carol   Subject: Mom

Alvin called to tell me Mom had a doctor's appointment today that I didn't have on my calendar. I decided not to cancel the appointment, and we arrived with no problems. I told the doctor she had a cold, and he kept probing. He had her get an X-ray, and she has bronchitis and a sinus infection. He gave her three prescriptions.

Other than that, she's doing well.

If I was scheduled to take our mother to the appointment, I blocked out enough time to travel to and from Mom's residence, to and from the doctor, and time for the appointment. In most cases, I took a half-day of vacation or I extended my workday. I allotted three to four vacation days a year for Mom's medical appointments and hospitalizations.

Three-Ring Binder

Mike brought a three-ring binder on his visits. It contained information for our mother such as insurance information, medications, contact information, directions, and emails on items he may encounter.

Labels

I used many labels for my mother. It takes time to create these labels, but once the template is created it is easy to copy another page when needed. I used them:

- To label Mom's medication in large print
- To provide required information (name, ID number, and date of birth) on the back of new prescriptions sent to her mail-order pharmacy
- For return address labels and to address holiday cards

Emergency Supplies

I kept a container of extra supplies in the car, including toiletry refills, a brush, pajamas, and a toothbrush. I hid backup items in her room. This ensured I could find items when I needed them. I also kept in my car a permanent marker for new clothing, medication labels, a small blanket for warmth, and snacks and bottled water in case a medical appointment was longer than expected.

These tools helped my brothers and me tremendously. The things-to-do list and visit summary were great tools to keep us focused on the priorities. The other tools enabled us to quickly retrieve information to organize our caregiving responsibilities. All of the tools helped make the journey less stressful.

 CHECKLIST

_____ Maintain a things-to-do list with the person responsible and a completion date for time sensitive items.

_____ Develop a list of your loved one's medications and medical providers.

_____ List items that continuously cause stress and identify ways to improve the situation.

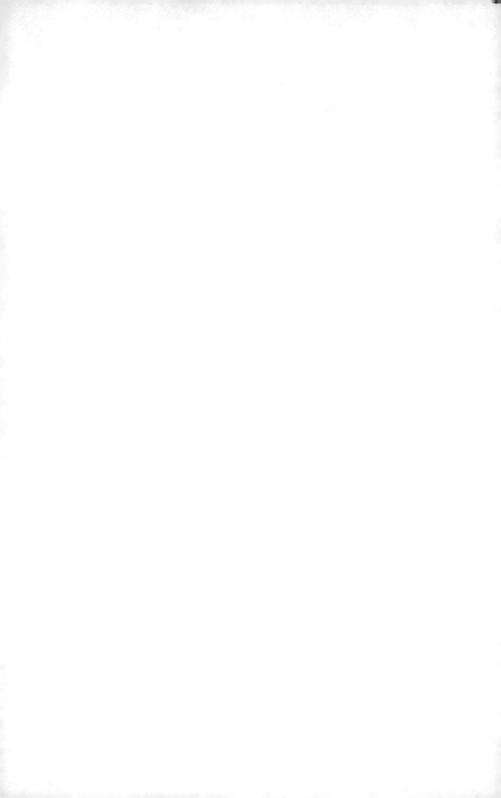

Chapter 16

Legal Affairs

• • • •

It is impossible to manage someone's affairs without the proper authority. For instance, my mother's hospital billed her for the $250 co-pay for a $62,829.41 hospitalization. I knew Mom owed $250, but I wanted to review the main components of the bill. I believed it was my responsibility to verify charges her insurance and/or Medicare paid on Mom's behalf. Although I had the summary bill, the hospital refused to send a detailed bill to my mother or me without my providing the power of attorney. These policies attempt to protect the person's privacy but make life more difficult for honest caregivers.

It was imperative for my brothers and me to have the legal documentation to carry out the affairs of our mother. Consult with a lawyer early to decide what multiple legal documents are needed to manage your loved one's affairs. These documents need to be executed when the person with Alzheimer's is in the early stages of the disease or before. Where possible, these documents should designate a primary and an alternate person. Basic definitions of these documents from the Alzheimer's Association website are below:

- "A **power of attorney** document allows a person with dementia (the principal) to name another individual (an agent or attorney-in-fact)—usually a spouse, domestic partner, trusted family member or friend—to make financial and other important decisions once the person with dementia no longer can."
- "A **guardian or conservator** is appointed by a court to make decisions about a person's care and property. Guardianship is generally considered when a person with dementia is no longer able to provide for his or her own care, and either the family is unable to agree upon the type of care needed or there is no family."
- Advanced Directives
  - > "A **power of attorney for health care** allows a person with dementia to name an agent to make health care-related decisions on his or her behalf when he or she is incapable of doing so. These decisions include choosing:
    - Doctors and other health care providers.
    - Types of treatments.
    - Care facilities."
  - > "A **living will** is a document that expresses how a physically or mentally incapacitated person wishes to be treated in certain medical situations. In a living will the person may state, among other things, his or her wishes regarding artificial life support. This document generally comes into play once a doctor decides that a person is incapacitated and unable to communicate his or her desires regarding life-sustaining treatment."
- "A **will** is a document identifying whom a person has chosen as:
  - > Executor: The person who will manage the estate.
  - > Beneficiaries: The people who will receive the assets in the estate."

- "A **living trust** is another way for the person to give instructions for how his or her estate should be handled upon death."
- "DNR: **Do-not-resuscitate**; refers to a person's instructions that, if his or her heart or breathing stops, the doctor should not try to restart it. A DNR is a medical instruction or order and must be issued by a physician." [1]

It is important to know the ownership and beneficiaries of assets such as a bank account, IRAs, and the like. This ownership and beneficiary designation for specific assets overrides distribution information in the will. Determine the beneficiaries of life insurance policies and social security benefits.

Some banks, hospitals, or doctors allow loved ones to give caregivers permission to handle his or her affairs. For example, I was the "patient representative" for my mother's mail-order pharmacy. These forms are only valid at that institution. While these forms are useful while executing the power of attorney and health care proxy documents, they should not be a substitute for the universal documents.

Advanced directives, living wills, and power of attorney for health care dictate the medical treatment the person will receive if incapacitated. It is good to have a discussion, if appropriate, to truly understand the wishes of the loved one. My mother discussed a high profile end-of-life case with me decades ago that helped me understand her wishes at that time. Because I believe advanced directives leave much to interpretation, I never shared these documents with medical professionals unless we felt the documents were needed.

Mike and I did not issue a do-not-resuscitate order for our mother until she was placed in hospice the last four days of her life. She had a good quality of life. Even when she was hospitalized, she was physically comfortable, although sometimes agitated. She enjoyed people, watching television, and a good laugh. She had more good days than bad even though she had three hospital stays and a rehabilitation stay totaling seven weeks the last four months of her life.

To: Mike   Date: 5/1/12

From: Carol   Subject: For you only

Mom's doctor asked if things start to go south, do we want to resuscitate. I said yes, but I would discuss with you. He doesn't think she will get to that point, but he wanted to ask. We may want to revisit our decision after your visit in July. It probably depends on her baseline quality of life.

Executing these legal documents is not always easy. The person is essentially transferring control of his or her life, health, and assets to another. It basically comes down to trust. Who does the loved one trust? My mother's generation believed men should manage legal and financial matters. I suggested to a friend her father might be more amenable to signing legal documents if her father's brother was involved.

Once these documents are signed and executed, make copies for appropriate family members and keep the originals in a safe place. A bank safety deposit box may not be a good place if family members cannot quickly retrieve the original documents.

The State of Delaware established a free legal advice hotline for seniors sixty years of age and above. The program aims to ensure the rights and financial security of seniors and is funded by a federal grant. Similar resources may be available in other states.

My mother's lawyer updated Mom's documents in 2004. Although the documents are not complicated, a reputable elder law firm is recommended. These documents must be correct because there may not be an opportunity to change them if your loved one's condition deteriorates. Ten years after Mom's power of attorney was executed, a financial institution questioned the completeness of the document. I located the law firm, but they had merged with another firm. I resolved the issue without involving the law firm. Mom's power of attorney had a list of ten powers she was granting. After each of the nine powers was a semicolon. After the last power, which happened to be at the bottom of a page was a period. The financial institution interpreted the period as a semicolon and believed the document was incomplete. I was able to point out that the period indicated there was no gap in the document.

Photo ID is now required for most medical appointments. My mother's Ohio identification card expired in January 2009. I wanted Mom to have another form of identification other than her passport. A tremendous amount of documentation was required to secure the Delaware identification card.

No time is good to think about final funeral arrangements for your loved one. If your loved one brings it up, listen to his or her wishes. If it appears appropriate, ask the loved one about his or her final wishes.

Proper documentation and authority are required to manage the health and financial affairs of loved ones. Execute these documents while your loved one is still able to communicate and execute his or her wishes.

 CHECKLIST

_____ Discuss wills, power of attorney, and a health care proxy with your loved one early.

_____ Take your loved one to a lawyer to execute his or her decisions with the proper legal documents. Make copies. Keep originals in a safe place.

_____ Have your loved one discuss his or her wishes with appropriate family members.

_____ Understand the ownership and beneficiaries of accounts and beneficiaries of insurance policies.

_____ Consider pre-need planning for funeral or final arrangements.

Part V

Meeting Needs in Different Residential Settings

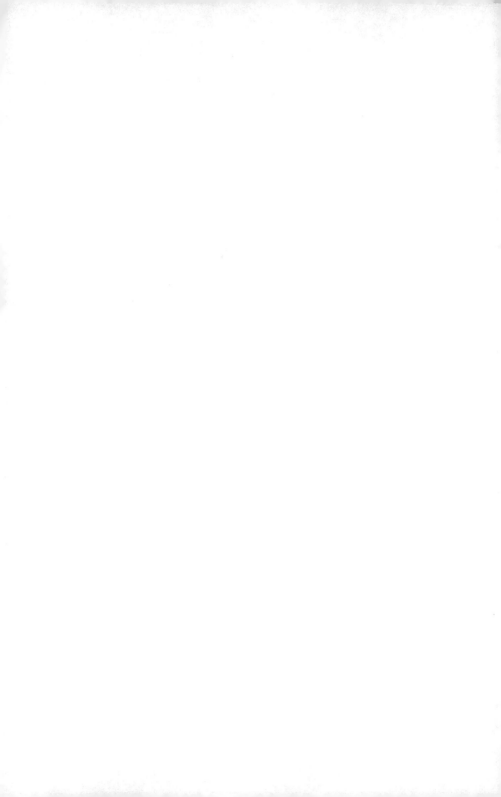

Chapter 17

Preparation for the Next Move

• • • •

I attended a great Alzheimer's Association event for caregivers. It included caregiver pampering, resource booths, and a fabulous meal. A family caregiver shared her story. She had vowed never to put her mother in a "home." By the end of her presentation, she said she had reluctantly placed her mother in a nursing home. It is difficult to provide around-the-clock long-term care for a person with Alzheimer's. My brothers and I knew the day would come when we would have to make a move, the day when our mother needed more care than we could provide.

The Caregiving Principle™, introduced in chapter 4, states:
Needs of the Person – Needs Filled by the Person =
Needs to Be Filled by the Caregiver(s).
Caregivers must provide those needs a person with Alzheimer's disease cannot provide for himself. Alzheimer's and age continually reduce the capability of a person to function, so caregivers must prepare in advance for the next move. The next move could be receiving more help from relatives or friends, using professional caregiver services, or moving the person to a facility. This chapter includes cost and funding information for care services and facilities and tools for selecting a facility.

Cost of Care

Keeping a person with Alzheimer's disease in a personal residence is usually the most cost-effective option, even if professional caregivers supplement the care. As more caregiving is needed, more professional caregiver help may be needed, and the cost increases. Professional homemakers provide a wide range of services including light housekeeping, meal preparation, changing beds, laundry, and shopping. Home health aides provide help with activities of daily living and monitor or administer medication. Some home health aides may perform some of the duties of a homemaker. Table 4 shows the 2017 cost of professional caregiving in states throughout the United States. Professional caregivers such as homemaker services and home health aides cost $131/day and $135/day respectively. These rates are based on annual rates and represent seven to eight hours of care a day. The median cost of adult day care is $70/day. The median base cost of an assisted-living facility is $3,750/month, but this excludes services such as medication administration or Alzheimer's care. The median cost of a nursing home semi-private room is $7,148/month. A person could require care in a facility for multiple years. One month of base cost assisted living is equivalent to twenty-eight days of home health aides. Understanding the residential costs helped us put in perspective the professional services we used for our mother. Costs for other areas of the country can be found on the Genworth Financial website.[1]

Table 4[2]

Long-Term Care Cost

	Median Monthly Nursing Home Rate: Private	Median Monthly Nursing Home Rate: Semi-Private	Median Monthly Assisted Living Base Rate Private	Median Home Health Aide Daily Rate	Median Home-maker Services Daily Rate	Median Adult Day Health Services Daily Rate
California	9703	8114	4275	157	157	77
Delaware	10996	10646	6015	139	138	73
Florida	8882	7908	3100	125	121	65
Kansas	6167	5551	4250	132	125	75
Louisiana	5475	5171	3293	96	94	63
Massachusetts	12471	11710	5599	163	158	65
New York	11701	11076	3988	149	141	80
Ohio	7604	6798	4178	133	132	57
United States	8121	7148	3750	135	131	70

Table 5 shows the residential care options for persons with Alzheimer's and how the costs are paid. Fifty-eight to 70 percent of persons with Alzheimer's live in a personal residence (their home or the home of a family member or friend). The current living arrangement, financial situation, and insurance benefits of the person with Alzheimer's will dictate the professional care options selected. Sources of funding for long-term care expenses are:

- *Personal funds.* Personal funds are used to pay for home aides, adult day care, assisted living facilities, memory care facilities, and nursing homes. Understand the financial situation of your loved one, including assets, debts, and income (pensions, Social Security, dividends, etc.).

- *Government programs.* Some states offer financial help for home health aides and assisted living to delay nursing home costs.[3] Most assisted-living facilities and memory care facilities not associated with a nursing home may not accept Medicare or Medicaid.

  › Medicare pays for short-term skilled nursing or rehabilitation care resulting from an illness or injury requiring a minimum three-night hospitalization. Medicare then pays one hundred percent for the first twenty days of a skilled nursing home or rehabilitation facility. For days twenty-one to one hundred, the patient pays in 2017 a copay of $164.50 each day. Private insurance or Medicaid may cover copays. After day one hundred, payment must be made by personal funds or covered by Medicaid. Medicare pays for the cost of hospice in a residence or facility.[4]

  › Medicaid will pay nursing home costs once the person meets the eligibility requirements by essentially exhausting most of his or her financial resources. Visit a Medicaid office and start the application process early to prevent delays.[5] Not all nursing homes accept Medicaid. Medicaid pays for the cost of hospice in a residence or facility.[6]

Table 5

Residential Caregiving Options

	PERSONAL RESIDENCE	ASSISTED LIVING	MEMORY CARE	NURSING HOME	HOSPICE FACILITY
HOUSING OPTIONS	58-70% [7,8]	4-10% [9]	2% [10]	15-20% [11]	2-4% [12,13]
AVERAGE U.S. COST	Typically lowest cost option	$45,000/ year median base rate, private ($123/ day) [14]	$56,772/ year ($156/ day) [15,16]	$82,128/ year semi-private ($225/ day) [17]	$238,079/ year ($652/ day) [18]
PAYMENT OPTIONS [19,20]	Long-Term Care Insurance, Private Pay, Medicaid (Limited), Veterans' Benefits	Long-Term Care Insurance, Private Pay, Medicaid (Limited)	Long-Term Care Insurance, Private Pay, Medicaid (Limited)	Long-Term Care Insurance, Private Pay, Medicare (Limited), Medicaid	Health Insurance, Medicare, Medicaid

- *Health Insurance.* Some health insurance policies pay for home care, short-term skilled nursing care, and hospice.
- *Long-term care insurance.* Long-term care insurance benefits begin when the person cannot perform at least two ADLs or when the person is cognitively impaired by any form of dementia. Long-term care policies pay a specified benefit daily, for a specified period, which may only cover some of your cost. Speak to a representative, and before ending your call ask, "What else should I know about this policy?" Most long-term care insurance policies can be used for home aides, adult day care, assisted living, memory care facilities, and nursing homes.

Providing long-term care for persons with Alzheimer's is expensive because the person can live with the disease for five, ten, or more years. Even a person with resources like a $200,000 house and $150,000 in savings can quickly deplete his or her resources if they are placed in a facility. Caregivers must use the money wisely and may have to liquidate a loved one's assets to pay for long-term care. Consult with a financial advisor because tax and other implications could be based on when and what assets are liquidated.

Selecting a Facility

Many times, care changes and moves are prompted at an inconvenient time for caregivers. Starting the search before needing a professional caregiver or facility allows a more leisurely and exhaustive search. Most facilities have websites that discuss the offerings. It is important to select the right kind of facility. For instance, a friend placed her father in an assisted-living facility, but he needed more skilled nursing care. So she moved him to a nursing home. Another friend placed his father in a nursing home, but they kept him too sedated so they moved him to assisted living. Try to minimize transition, which causes stress both to the loved one and the family.

Selecting a facility takes time. The Alzheimer's Association can provide a list of facilities in your area. When my brothers moved our mother to an assisted-living facility, we did not conduct an extensive search of facilities but relied on a visit Mike made in January 2004.

To: Carol, Ron   Date: 1/16/04

From: Mike   Subject: Assisted-Living Facility

I mailed to you today information on an assisted living senior community. I have begun investigating assisted-living facilities to get a feel for what is out there (that is, type of facility, location, cost, level of care, etc.) in the event this is something Mom may need in the future. The scary thing is the waiting list to get into these facilities can be long. I was pleasantly surprised to find the current waiting list is only about two months.

I first heard of the facility from a member of our church in Cincinnati who moved her father from his home to this facility. I then found this is one of a few assisted-living facilities located in Mom's area.

Our focus should be to continue to do what we can to keep Mom living in her house. Knowing the monthly cost of an assisted-living facility will be helpful to put in perspective the extra costs associated with keeping Mom in her home (that is, social worker, nurse). It should always be cheaper for Mom to stay in her own home unless she reaches the need for skilled nursing home care.

Eight months later, when it was time to act, I quickly retrieved the information Mike sent and alerted the facility about my brother's visit.

One year later my brothers and I used a systematic method to evaluate both assisted-living and memory care facilities in Delaware. We wanted a facility that could meet Mom's needs as she continued to decline. We received a list of facilities from the Alzheimer's Association and from a work-life balance resource my employer provided. The Alzheimer's Association website has a care facility checklist.[21] We created a spreadsheet to collect and compare the data on the following for each facility:

- Name, website URL
- Cost
- Medication (facility or family supplies)
- Move-in requirements (TB test, medical evaluation, etc.)

- Security to prevent wandering outside the facility
- Availability of rooms
- Room size
- Number of residents in a room
- Bathing facilities (in room vs. shared)
- Odors
- Room amenities (furnishings, phone, cable, etc.)
- Carpeting compared with tile floors
- Daily program
- Outside trips (scenic drives, shopping, etc.)
- Distance from my home and place of work
- General comments (demeanor of residents and staff)
- Diversity of residents (visual)

Mike and I collected the information and shared the spreadsheet and pictures with Ron. We deliberated, asked the staff follow-up questions, and collectively selected a memory care facility.

The same approach can be used for nursing home evaluation and selection. A source of nursing home ratings is www.cms.gov.[22] This website contains useful information on Medicaid and Medicare services. Another source of nursing home ratings is the *U.S. News and World Report*.[23] Speak to family, friends, and colleagues about their experiences with nursing homes. Have them share their issues, concerns, and selection criteria. Develop selection criteria for evaluating nursing homes. Visit the recommended nursing homes and others. Ratings are a starting point to identify nursing homes so visit the facility multiple times to make a good personal assessment.

Starting the search early may give options on room size, number of roommates, view, and other details. Starting the search too late may lead to having to place a loved one in the only nursing home and room available. Most nursing homes have a waiting list. Caregivers should place their loved one on the waiting list for their top two to three nursing homes. When there is an opening, caregivers should honestly assess the loved one's condition and consider if it is the right time for a move.

This section of the book, "Meeting Needs in Different Residential Settings," discusses how caregivers with the support of others can meet the needs of persons with Alzheimer's. Our personal experiences and decisions are shared. Some advice for moving a person to a facility:

- Caregivers should spend quality time selecting the facility. Make sure it is the right type of facility. Visit the desired facility multiple times during different times of the day (mealtimes, activity time, evening).

- Caregivers should conduct research by speaking with others who have experience with the facility.

- Caregivers should get to know the staff and aides to keep the lines of communication open. If I was near my mother's memory care after returning from a late trip or social activity, I stopped in. This allowed me to interact with the night staff and observe my mother during the late hours.

- Caregivers should be involved with the loved one's care to ensure that he or she receives consistent and proper care. Be there as much as possible. Do not be afraid to politely ask questions or convey concerns you have. Use the proper chain of command to report concerns and be open to their recommendations. Make sure you understand their plan to address your concern.

- Caregivers should recognize there will be an adjustment period for the loved one and caregiver.

It is easy to anticipate the next level of care needed, but it is more difficult to predict when. Early option evaluation and preliminary selection of professional caregivers and facilities can reduce the anxiety once these resources are needed.

The primary residence is the most cost-effective housing option for persons with Alzheimer's. Caregivers can supplement care with family and professional caregivers. The cost of facility care can be significant and varies from state-to-state. Caregivers must consider type and cost when selecting a place. Facility checklists, ratings information, and information from family and friends can help caregivers make the correct choice.

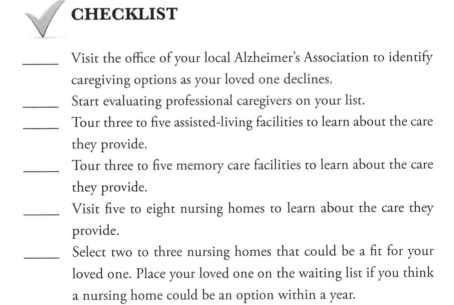 **CHECKLIST**

_____ Visit the office of your local Alzheimer's Association to identify caregiving options as your loved one declines.

_____ Start evaluating professional caregivers on your list.

_____ Tour three to five assisted-living facilities to learn about the care they provide.

_____ Tour three to five memory care facilities to learn about the care they provide.

_____ Visit five to eight nursing homes to learn about the care they provide.

_____ Select two to three nursing homes that could be a fit for your loved one. Place your loved one on the waiting list if you think a nursing home could be an option within a year.

Chapter 18

Caregiving in the Personal Residence

• • • •

Our mother lived alone in her home as she began to exhibit signs of Alzheimer's disease. My brothers and I were usually never physically there when issues arose, so we never knew if an event occurred as she explained. At times, however, we were there and witnessed the same events, but they happened differently in Mom's mind. We wanted her to remain in her home as long as possible, but we wondered if we were doing the right thing. Eventually Mom demonstrated she could not live alone.

Many cases of Alzheimer's disease are diagnosed while a person is living in a personal residence. Family members and friends will notice changes in the person's behavior. These warning signs should prompt family members to investigate the situation and get a diagnosis (chapter 3, A Watchful Eye). A diagnosis of Alzheimer's is devastating. Openly discuss the diagnosis with your loved one and listen to what he or she says. Be empathetic and provide reassurance that he or she will be taken care of.

Observe how your loved one manages his or her ADLs and IADLs. Speak with family members who will have a major role in the care of the person (chapter 2, Circle of Support). Unless there is a safety issue, caregivers should not make rash decisions about caring for their loved one. If medication is prescribed, wait for the medication to stabilize. Make the current environment safe, even if other housing situations are being considered. Learn about Alzheimer's disease using the resources discussed in chapter 13 and speak to others who are caring for a person with the illness.

Develop a plan. This plan may begin as a skeleton as you pursue multiple issues simultaneously such as:

- Medical – Testing may be necessary for a better diagnosis or for other medical issues.
- Financial – Gain understanding of the person's resources, assets, and debts.
- Legal – Execute legal documents (chapter 16, Legal Affairs) to obtain information and authority to execute the plan.
- Create your circle of support. Find out who can help and how.

The plan must consider the specific circumstances of the person with Alzheimer's. There may be no support network or a support network all around. The plan does not have to be finished or cast in stone. As the above issues are explored, the plan may change and then finally crystallize.

Multiple living arrangements are available for persons with Alzheimer's. The most convenient place, in the early stages, is a personal residence. Fifty-eight percent of persons with Alzheimer's are living in a personal residence.[1] The advantages of remaining in a personal residence are:

- The person is familiar with the residence and initially can perform his or her ADLs and some IADLs. The familiarity will give him or her a sense of security.
- The disruption to the lifestyle is minimized.
- The person is familiar with the neighborhood.
- Neighbors or local agencies may be able to provide some caregiving support.
- The person can continue some of his or her social activities in the community (golf, garden club, church, etc.).
- The residence is usually the most cost-effective scenario for persons with Alzheimer's.

The person should not live alone unless adequate and consistent support is present. If the plan moves the person to another personal residence, a transition could take months.

Caregivers for a person with Alzheimer's living at home must reach out for help. They have an extremely challenging task that eventually becomes an around-the-clock responsibility. As the disease progresses, the caregiver spends a greater part of the time with ADLs. Caregivers should learn about the disease and personal care to reduce some of the stress. The Alzheimer's Association offers caregiving training courses online and in person. Many families attend workshops together so everyone receives the training. Caregivers should participate in Alzheimer's support groups to learn from other caregivers. Three good resources for family members providing daily care for a person with Alzheimer's are:

- *Personal Care: Assisting a Person with Middle- or Late-Stage Dementia with Daily Needs,* Alzheimer's Association, rev. Dec. 16, 770-10-00191.[2]

- *The 36-Hour Day: A Family Guide to Caring for People Who Have Alzheimer's Disease, Related Dementias, and Memory* by Nancy L. Mace and Peter V. Rabins.[3]
- EssentiALZ®, online dementia training from Alzheimer's Association and HealthCare Interactive Inc. Offers six courses including one on activities of daily living.[4]

Caregivers can utilize adult day care for persons who should not be alone while family members are working. These centers vary greatly by the focus of activities and the services they provide. Some adult day care centers focus on persons with Alzheimer's disease.[5] Caregivers can work with the staff to ensure the center is a good fit for the loved one. Adult day care can provide a break for full-time caregivers.

Caregivers need to establish a daily routine for the person with Alzheimer's. The routine should include items to meet the physiological and some social needs. Set waking times, meal times, bath times, and bed times, and add household chores and activities for the remainder of the day. Challenging tasks should be reserved for the morning when the person is most alert.

In the early phase of the disease, most persons can meet most of the physiological need (chapter 5). As the disease progresses, the amount of caregiving will increase. Caregivers can seek the help of professional caregivers, such as home aides, home health aides, social workers, case managers, and nurses. They are a great resource because most have Alzheimer's experience and can tailor advice to specific situations. Home aides are usually not certified but perform services such as housekeeping, laundry, meal preparation, and companionship.[6] Home health aides are certified and help with personal care (ADLs), medications, and medical monitoring. Nurses are certified and provide skilled nursing care. Social workers and care managers help assess the needs and recommend resources and professionals such as a speech therapist.[7]

Professional caregivers can tailor their service by helping on a monthly, weekly, or daily basis. Seek out recommendations. There are self-employed caregivers and caregivers from agencies. Most caregiving agencies will visit, assess the needs, and then recommend the right kind of caregiver(s).

Family caregivers will experience physical demands. They may need to help the loved one stand, walk, navigate stairs, and get in and out of the car. To avoid injury, correct techniques should be learned and used.

The safety need can be met in the personal residence. The person will have his or her sense of safety need met by being surrounded by familiar people, furnishings, and scents. The residence must be safe, though, so caregivers do not have to watch the person continuously. Chapter 6, Safety Need, helps caregivers make the home safe. As the illness progresses, more precautions may be needed to maintain a safe environment.

The social need can be met in a personal residence if the loved one continues to participate in some of his or her current hobbies. An hour or so organizing baseball cards, selecting yarn for a knitting project, or hitting golf balls in the backyard may be engaging as well. He or she may not be able to play bridge but may enjoy watching friends play. Social interactions with neighbors, the mail carrier, newspaper carrier, and regular visitors to the neighborhood can also meet the social need. Periodically identify opportunities outside the home (chapter 7, Social Need). The weekend section of the newspaper lists many options.

Avoid activities the person is unable to do or that could cause frustration. Periodically reassess his or her capability to participate in these activities. Activities a person with Alzheimer's disease can manage safely today may become a hazard tomorrow. Activities involving judgment or potentially dangerous tools or those that could lead to a harmful situation should be discontinued.

The esteem need can be met in a personal residence. The esteem is determined by what he or she contributes and how he or she is treated.

Providing opportunities for the person to contribute to the household, family, community, and church can help meet the need for esteem. Treating a person with dignity and respect will also maintain his or her esteem (chapter 8, Esteem Need).

Caregiving in a personal residence is extremely challenging. The behaviors a person with Alzheimer's exhibits can be very stressful. While interacting with our mother, my brothers and I carefully chose our battles. Knowing when to let go is important. Regardless of how understanding and compassionate I tried to be, sometimes I said or did the wrong thing. When this happened, I apologized and gave Mom a hug immediately. The Alzheimer's Association understands the stress, frustration, and difficulty of caring for a person with the disease so they provide a twenty-four-hour hotline to assist caregivers involved with challenging situations. The number is 1-800-272-3900.[8]

My brothers and I were caregivers from a distance when our mother lived in her home with early signs of Alzheimer's disease. My family reached out to professionals (doctors, social workers, and a nurse) for help. We could not completely meet Mom's needs from a distance and eventually moved her.

Caregivers can meet the needs of a loved one living together in a personal residence, but it is a very challenging role. Caregivers must learn about the disease and proper care. They should reach out for help from their circle of support. They can augment the care with professional caregivers to ensure that the needs of the loved one are met and to reduce the stress of caregiving.

CHECKLIST

_____ Obtain the recommended reference material.

_____ Prepare a caregiving plan for your loved one with a contingency plan for caregiver or weather emergencies.

_____ Create your circle of support with those who can assist and list the services they can provide.

Chapter 19

I Never Thought She Would…

• • • •

*When I told a friend I was going to Cleveland to move my
mother to assisted living, she replied in sort of a cold way, saying,
"What did she almost burn down?" What my friend was really
saying is it takes a drastic event for family to realize the severity
of the situation. The event may lead to the loss of property
(house, car, or money), but oftentimes these same events could have
caused the death of the loved one and/or others.*

Older persons with mild cognitive impairment (MCI) have
an increased risk of developing dementia.[1] The transition
from MCI to Alzheimer's is not easy to predict. Often, a
defining moment on this Alzheimer's journey occurs when the family
realizes their loved one has more than MCI and can no longer function
properly. Maybe the family decides the person should not drive, cook,
or live safely in the current circumstance. Family members say, "I never
thought she/he would…," but they did, and they will do it again if no
one intervenes. Our defining moment helped us realize Mom could no
longer live alone.

To: Carol, Ron   Date: 8/31/04

From: Mike   Subject: Today's Incident

I received a call from the police tonight at a little past 9:00 p.m. Mom called the police because of the following incident. Supposedly she was willingly picked up at home by three people she did not know and driven around. As they got to the bank she refused to go in, but one of the males did go in. Mom reported she is missing a check she wrote to herself for $5,000, her black purse, and all of her identification. The officer called me while at Mom's. He is filing a police report and will check with the bank tomorrow. He said her checking records were not good so he could not tell if a check was missing.

I called Mom again after talking with Carol. Mom did find her purse and identification. I informed the police. I spoke to the officer who investigated the incident, and he said Mom had written on a sheet of paper "two young ladies have me in a snare. I think they have $5,000 of mine." This may be what Mom wrote prior to calling the police.

Carol and I don't think this incident occurred. Sounds familiar?

Next steps:

- Officer will call the bank to check on transactions in the morning. Carol may have to call since she is on this account.
- Carol informed Mom's sister tonight. Mom's sister will visit Mom as part of her regular Wednesday visit.
- Mike will make an appointment with her new doctor within two weeks to see if she can be prescribed a drug to deal with these "dreams" or "hallucinations." Carol will follow up with a pre-visit letter to her doctor. Mike will be there for doctor's visit.

- Carol will inform the social worker of the situation for guidance.
- Carol to ask Mom to check her purse(s) to see if she can find the check.
- We don't know if the police will contact a social services agency regarding this incident.

To: Carol, Mike   Date: 9/2/04

From: Ron   Subject: (No Subject)

The so-called house break-in was about her financial papers. Look at the bank incidents of two men taking her money and the bank taking her money to operate the bank. And now this. If these calls continue, the police may consider taking Mom to a hospital for observation as being "gravely disabled."

I get the impression Mom is frequently checking certificates of deposit rates to move money to get the highest rate. It seems that financial security bothers her, and maybe it's time you take some of this control from her.

I haven't called regarding this incident in order to get as much information on the matter first. Did the police actually catch someone? How did they get her into the car? Why would she go with them? Was anyone actually arrested?

Any consideration to making Mom aware she is experiencing these dreams? If it were true she would have been hurt, her car may have been stolen, house ransacked, and purse and other items taken.

Regarding your trip, all I can recommend is to tie in her accounts and see if she would be receptive to freezing some of her funds for her protection. Maybe the bank would have to contact one of you before it could be touched. This may make her feel more comfortable. Just a thought.

Medically, every couple of months an issue arises, and this is the second one with the police. What is the detective's opinion on this incident? We could be getting close to assisted living!!!!!

The "incident" was not a delusion or a dream. It was all too real. Alzheimer's will result in uncharacteristic behavior. My brothers and I were grateful Mom was not harmed. We were blessed God had His arms of protection around her. We do not know what happened, and we never will. **I never thought she would** give away five thousand dollars of her hard-earned money to strangers...but she did. This was our "defining moment" or our "enough is enough" or our "wake-up call." We had worked hard during the last two years to help Mom maintain her independence. Now we knew, without a shadow of a doubt, that she could not live on her own.

Taking responsibility for our mother was extremely hard, but my brothers and I had no other choice. Mom was a strong woman, with a strong work ethic and a strong faith in God. I always depended on her strength and decisiveness, even if I did not always agree with her. Now my brothers and I were making major decisions on her behalf. We knew that moving Mom to assisted living was the right decision, but it was physically and mentally draining.

Alzheimer's disease can be baffling and results in uncharacteristic behaviors and action. The family will say, "I never thought she/he would...." It is difficult to predict the uncharacteristic act that will become your defining moment. But do not wait for it to happen before you act. Keep your loved one out of danger by taking action sooner rather than later. Think about stopping him or her from driving, disconnecting the stove, eliminating access to bank accounts and credit cards, and placing alarms on doors. In short, do whatever you have to do to keep him or her safe.

 ## CHECKLIST

_____ Provide adequate supervision for the person with MCI or Alzheimer's.

_____ Think about what you can do to prevent your loved one from having a "defining moment."

Chapter 20

Caregiving in the Assisted-Living Facility

• • • •

I believed that moving our mother out of her home would be devastating for her...the beginning of the end. The situation was quite the contrary. Although Mom tried to return home multiple times, her home had become more of a burden than a joy. She did not miss maintaining a house and yard, paying bills, or purchasing and cooking food. Mild cognitive impairment made these tasks more difficult. Mom felt a great sense of relief when assisted living reduced her responsibilities.

I was proud of how Mike took charge when we discovered we needed to change our mother's living situation. He conveyed four or five things he was planning to do including taking Mom to Cincinnati the next day. I asked, "Then what?" And he replied in such a definitive way, "I don't know!" What he was doing was removing Mom from a potentially dangerous situation so the family could focus on developing a plan.

My brothers and I had to decide what kind of housing (living with a family member, assisted living, or nursing home) and where (Cleveland, southern Ohio—near Mike, or Delaware—near me). She had always objected to moving in with my brother or me. She wanted her own place, she wanted her independence, and she did not want to be a burden on anyone. We felt she could receive care and remain independent in assisted living in Cleveland. This allowed her to continue her activities and associations with family, church family, and friends. After much thought and deliberation, our plan was to move her to an assisted-living facility in Cleveland.

To: Carol, Mike   Date: 9/9/04

From: Ron   Subject: (no subject)

The change Mom will be facing is tremendous, and it will be difficult for her to part with a lot of items. This is why storage is necessary. I think this is where we may have to bend a little. She will already be losing her house and car. I won't make any arrangements for storage until we have an idea of the space needed.

We will also have to monitor Mom's behavior for signs of depression.

My brothers and I converged on our mother's house for an "intervention," to persuade her to move to assisted living. Two of her sisters joined us. We purposely scheduled the meeting for the morning when Mom was most alert. We discussed each of our concerns, which were:

- Safety
- Health – weight under a hundred pounds
- Burdens of maintaining a house
- Minimal socialization

Our mother was receptive to touring the assisted-living facility, and she selected her apartment. After eating lunch there, Mom was completely sold on the idea. She immediately became concerned about the work involved with moving, but we assured her we would manage everything…and we did.

Assisted-living facilities bridge the gap between living independently and living in a nursing home. The facility supplies and maintains a room, suite, or apartment. Many facilities charge a daily base cost that may only include room, food, housekeeping, activities, and minimum resident support. Other items such as phone, cable, laundry, Alzheimer's care, medication administration, and transport to doctor visits may be an extra cost.[1] Often family members will supplement the care to ensure all needs of the resident are met. The federal government does not regulate assisted living.[2]

A large variation exists in assisted-living facilities, so it's important to understand the services provided. Caregivers should read the facility's marketing and contract information carefully and understand the total cost and projected future cost as the person declines. An application fee may be required, but in many cases, they do not require a long-term lease. Caregivers should anticipate how the loved one will receive and adapt to the change. Evaluate how to lessen the impact of the changes. For instance, if the loved one is accustomed to dinner at 7 p.m., but the facility serves dinner at 5 p.m. and 6 p.m., requesting a 6 p.m. dinnertime will be less of a change. Caregivers can develop a list of items (schedule, policies, etc.) that may become an issue and identify how these potential issues will be managed.

Living in an assisted-living facility helped meet our mother's physiological need. The facility supplied a spacious apartment with a living area, kitchenette, bedroom, and bathroom. My brothers and I made her apartment homelike and comfortable with familiar items from her home including family pictures. Assisted living provided three healthy and tasty meals (and snacks) a day, and Mom began to gain weight. The clinical staff administered Mom's medication.

The assisted-living facility was a safe environment by design. They have elevators, emergency call buttons, safety bars in the bathrooms, and the watchful eyes of staff members. Our mother was safe and secure, but the assisted-living facility did not meet her sense of security because she was not at home. She constantly tried to leave and go home.

To: Ron, Carol   Date: 10/10/04

From: Mike   Subject: Mom's on Observation

Not sure if you are aware, but Mom was placed on observation. She is not to leave the building. During the day someone is to check on her every couple of hours. Carol found this out when she called Sunday afternoon.

The reason for this is Mom was in the parking lot Sunday morning trying either to get a ride or to get a car to go somewhere. I am a bit confused as to what she was trying to do. She also did not understand she now lives in assisted living.

Mom is in much worse shape than we thought.

Very mentally draining.

My brothers and I were hopeful the assisted-living facility would allow our mother to live fairly independently with minimal support, but the move was extremely eye opening. We did not realize how much the Alzheimer's disease had affected her since she had masked it. While in the assisted-living facility, she was quite disoriented at times and had difficulty remembering the location of her room or the names of her tablemates. The adjustment to assisted living took months compared with the days we had anticipated. Mom moved in on Saturday, and we left town on Monday. In retrospect, this was an inadequate transition period. We looked for help from her geriatric doctor.

To: Ron, Mike   Date: 10/20/04
From: Carol   Subject: Doctor call

The doctor is not concerned about Mom's behavior. He believes Mom is making the adjustment, just not as fast as we want. He believes the excess walking the halls is pent-up energy and we need to get her involved in the local activities. The dreams he called delusions, and he mentioned persons with Alzheimer's lose their sense of time. So if she said she went to the restaurant and couldn't find her car, it probably did happen at some time in her life. Misperception of her surroundings and events is common. His recommendation is to give her time, continue to reassure her, and constantly re-orient her to the new surroundings. I talked about her being anxious when we visit, and he said that's because we were changing her routine. He had an answer for everything...but I didn't feel he was trying to dismiss my concerns.

Time and increased participation in the facility's activities helped her make the adjustment and feel more at home.

Assisted living helped meet our mother's social need. She shared meals with three other residents and interacted with assisted living and independent living residents. They offered many activities, such as live music, ice cream socials, and Mom's favorite, Bingo. After breakfast she read the newspaper in the parlor with other residents.

Assisted living helped meet our mother's esteem need. She felt she was living independently, and the staff treated her with respect. She developed good relationships with the caregivers. Mom was glad she could still provide a place for us to stay (sleep sofa in her living area) when we visited.

To: Carol, Mike   Date: 11/2/04

From: Ron   Subject: (no subject)

Talked to Mom last night. She's very happy with assisted living. Really enjoys the food, no cooking, and no gardening. She said, "So this is what retirement is all about." She said she told the staff they'll have to drag her out to get rid of her.

I didn't say anything about her being on observation but re-emphasized not going out alone. She mentioned several times being glad she's not a burden to us. So I'm glad she still feels a sense of independence.

The Caregiving Principle™ states that caregivers must provide those needs of a person that he or she cannot provide for himself or herself. The caregiving role of my brothers and I changed when our mother moved to assisted living. We aided with her transition by meeting the staff and accepting the recommendations to ease her transition to a new way of life. Mike assumed responsibility for managing her finances, and my brothers and I managed her medical appointments. With the help of her assisted-living facility, we met most of Mom's needs and our needs as well. We had peace of mind knowing she was safe, eating, and taking her medications and was well cared for. If an issue came up, the staff could investigate. As the disease progressed, Mom began to get up at night to check that the doors to the facility were locked. She was not able to rest peacefully at night.

An assisted-living facility can meet the needs of someone with mild cognitive impairment or in the early phases of Alzheimer's disease. Residents are provided meals, living quarters, and social activities in a safe environment. The responsibility of the loved one is reduced. Family members know the loved one is cared for, and the staff monitors their loved one.

 CHECKLIST

_____ Tour three to five assisted-living facilities.

_____ If your loved one moves to an assisted-living facility, monitor the transition and the care he or she receives.

Chapter 21

Caregiving in the Memory Care Facility

• • • •

My brothers and I believed assisted living would be my mother's home for the next two to three years. Within a year, however, we and the staff were concerned about her leaving the facility at night. We had the option of moving her to a memory care facility on the same property. I felt the next transition should be closer to one of us. Assisted living was nice and met all of our goals. But anytime an issue arose, we were still handling the situation from a distance.

A memory care facility is designed (programs, activities) for the unique needs of persons with Alzheimer's. These facilities have a physical layout tailored and a staff specifically trained to manage the challenging Alzheimer's behaviors, such as confusion, sleep disturbances, desire to walk, and aggression. Memory care facilities offer educational programs and support groups for family members and are active in advocacy efforts in the Alzheimer's community.[1]

When my family began searching for a secure facility for our mother, these facilities were called Alzheimer's Special Care Units. The name sounded cold, closed, and isolated; but the facilities we visited were quite the opposite, so memory care is a more appropriate name.

If the memory care facility is large, the residents are often grouped into smaller sections, wings, or floors of the building. The residents may be grouped based on their capability. Each group usually has separate dining and living facilities with an area where all residents gather for events such as entertainment. The smaller groups promote a routine, consistency (same caregivers), familiarity, and a sense of community or family. My mother's memory care facility included twenty-two other residents. She did not know their names, but she recognized their faces. She once commented about a new resident, "I didn't know they let people eat here who don't live here."

Memory care facilities charge a base cost. Additional costs are based on how much care the person needs (ADL assistance, medication administration, etc.). As the person declines from Alzheimer's and other illnesses, the amount and cost of care increase.

Memory care is equipped to provide more of the ADLs than assisted living. More important, the staff is trained to understand and overcome the challenges of meeting the basic needs while keeping the anxiety level at a minimum.

Memory care meets the physical safety need of residents. They provide elevators, emergency call buttons, safety bars in the bathrooms, and the watchful eyes of staff members. These facilities are secure with locked or alarmed doors to eliminate wandering. Residents can walk in safe areas twenty-four hours a day. Not all residents understand they cannot leave. They may not have tried to leave, or they may not know the location of the exit. Initially, the resident will not have a sense of security because they are not home and the adjustment period can take months. Mom's adjustment took six to nine months. Some residents find comfort by believing they are on vacation, in a college dorm, or on a business trip.

Memory care meets the social need of residents with mentally stimulating activities geared to residents with Alzheimer's. If the memory care unit is part of a larger facility, the residents may interact with residents without the disease. They provide live entertainment, holiday celebrations, family nights, and trips out (country rides, sporting events, restaurants, etc.).

Memory care meets the esteem need of residents because caregivers treat each resident with dignity and respect. They maintain a focus on the emotional state of each resident. The residents can build esteem by contributing to the operation of the facility by setting the table or baking cookies, for example. Memory care meets the self-actualization need by helping residents function as independently as they can.

My brothers and I struggled with putting our mother in a secured facility. We felt we were putting her in jail and used terms such as "lock up" and "lock down" to describe these facilities. But we knew these facilities had the safeguards she needed. We could have moved her to a secure facility on the same property, but a transition is a transition if it is one mile or one hundred miles. Most of all, leaving Mom in a locked facility in Cleveland felt like abandonment.

My brothers and I also struggled with moving our mother from Cleveland to Delaware. At the time, we were not using The Caregiving Principle™. But we considered the change in Mom's social environment. Delaware would allow my regular visits, reduce the visits from Mike and his family, and almost eliminate visits from siblings, friends, and church members. We knew moving her to Delaware was a large concern of Mom's after living in the Cleveland area for more than sixty-five years. She mentioned if she moved she might not see her family or friends again. Unfortunately I knew she was right, but we felt it was more important for Mom to live close to one of her children.

To: Ron, Mike   Date: 9/22/05

From: Carol   Subject: Re: (no subject)

We need to proceed with moving Mom to Delaware. I believe it is the best thing for her. I personally think she will be ok with moving. If she accepts it right off, I wouldn't go into a lot of the rationale.

I believe we did the right thing by keeping Mom in Cleveland last year based on the information we had at the time. We believed she could still get around…but she was further along than we believed.

One of the worst days of my life was when Mom moved to Wilmington, Delaware, because the move never sank in. Upon arrival, Mom was livid about her new residence. The staff helped to calm her down by providing lunch and getting Mom settled in her room. I was on the front line, so I called for backup.

To: Ron, Carol   Date: 10/10/05

From: Mike   Subject: Mom's Initial Impressions

Around 3:30 p.m. Carol reported Mom was not happy in Delaware when she saw: (1) the location in a suburban or country setting, and (2) she only has the one bedroom and shared bathroom and sitting area. Keep in mind her furniture, pictures, etc., do not arrive until Saturday.

Although I was the strongest proponent of this move, I had 100 percent support of my brothers to make this move work. Mike was prepared to travel to Delaware if necessary.

Then Alvin walked in, and I smiled because I now had more help. But even more important Mom had a great big smile on her face. Eventually, the caregivers suggested that Alvin and I leave. I did not want to leave... but I was glad to leave. It had been a long, exhausting day.

The transition from assisted living to memory care was difficult. Mom was disoriented and constantly tried to leave and "go home." Eventually, she made the transition. I believe this transition was easier because:

- The memory care facility footprint was smaller. They had bedrooms for twenty-three residents, kitchen, dining room, patio, and multiple common areas all on one floor.
- The residents participated in activities appropriate for their ability all day.
- They had a higher staff-to-resident ratio than in her assisted-living facility.
- Many staff members have a passion to care for persons with Alzheimer's disease.
- My frequent visits reassured Mom.

To: Ron, Mike   Date: 5/7/06
From: Carol   Subject: Laundry

Mom called and wondered if I had taken some of her clothes. I mentioned they might be getting washed. It's good she is becoming more aware of things. I told her sometimes it's easier for her to deal with these issues in the day because she gets confused at night. She said, "I get confused during the day." I had to smile.

Mom received her candy from Ron on Saturday, and she offered a piece to the activities coordinator and some of the residents. The bottom line is she likes all the people there. As I left today, she patted her "friend" on the shoulder, and the friend smiled.

Mom likes to see me to the door. This is uncomfortable because I try to get to the door before her and unlock it. Then I give her a big hug with my leg holding the door open. A few times she said she would wait in the hallway until the elevator comes, but I tell her I'm taking the stairs.

The Caregiving Principle™ states that caregivers must provide those needs of the persons that they cannot provide for themselves. The role of my brothers and me changed when our mother moved to memory care in Delaware. I visited her regularly and could resolve issues immediately. I was her primary link to the outside world and took her to medical appointments, church worship services, and social activities. Initially she could perform her ADLs but needed assistance with all of them by the time she passed away eight-and-a-half years later. Her facility provided a suite, tasty and nutritious meals and snacks, clothes laundering, housekeeping, outings, and medication administration. It was a comfortable, safe, and secure environment with activities throughout the day. Mom participated in Bible study, lunch outings, musical performances, and holiday celebrations with the larger assisted living community. She set the table, folded laundry, and occasionally took the community dog out for a walk (with a caregiver). My mother felt she was living independently. She became an ambassador for her area. She befriended new residents and told them, "You will like it here." The staff loved Mom (or Mrs. Boyd, Ms. E., or Ms. Liz, as she was called) and boosted her esteem regularly. The residents and staff became her family. With time, the memory care facility became her home.

To: Mike   Date: 4/13/14
From: Carol   Subject: Re: Mom was scheduled to
                            leave hospital at 1 p.m.
Went back to Mom's facility. She was in her bed with a grin on her face watching "Wheel of Fortune" on her television. Mom knows she is home.

My family, with the help of her memory care facility, met the physiological, safety, social, esteem, and self-actualization needs of our mother. Periodically she talked about living in memory care. She mentioned how much she liked living there and took credit for finding and selecting it as her home. This was definitely one time when I took the expert's advice and did not correct her.

A memory care facility can meet the needs of residents through all stages of the disease. Residents are provided meals and rooms in a family-like atmosphere. They are safe and can walk in a secure environment. There are appropriate social activities and entertainment to keep residents engaged. In most cases, residents are treated with respect, and family members know the loved one is cared for and safe.

✓ CHECKLIST

_____ Tour three to five memory care facilities.

_____ If your loved one moves to a memory care facility, monitor the transition and the care he or she receives.

Chapter 22

Caregiving in the Nursing Home

• • • •

Our plan was to keep our mother in memory care as long as
possible. My brothers and I knew her health could decline to the
point that her memory care facility could no longer care for her.
To prepare for the next move, Mike and I visited nursing homes
multiple times and conducted a first-hand evaluation of the
rehabilitation facilities in which she stayed.

Nursing homes provide care to those recovering from an illness (short-term) or with chronic medical problems (long-term). Many are skilled nursing facilities (SNF) and cater to those who are temporarily or permanently incapacitated. A SNF provides medical, pharmacy, dietary, and twenty-four-hour nursing supervision and assistance with ADLs. Persons living in nursing homes must be under the care of the nursing home physician. Nursing facilities are licensed by the state and must comply with standards for care and services.[1] Many nursing homes have a section dedicated to the special needs of residents with Alzheimer's. Many nursing homes have updated the décor to a more residential appearance.

The resident pays nursing home fees until his or her resources are depleted. Residents will then use their monthly income, minus a $30-

to-$120 personal allowance, to pay for the nursing home. Medicaid will pay the rest.[2] Determine if the nursing home accepts Medicaid once your loved one runs out of money to avoid another transition when funds are depleted.

Placing a loved one in a nursing home can be emotional. Some caregivers promised they would never place their loved one in a nursing home but found that providing twenty-four-hour care was difficult. Caregivers may have feelings of premature loss or that they are abandoning their loved one. The person with Alzheimer's may have feelings of abandonment or may be coping with his or her own mortality. This can be a highly emotional and difficult time for everyone. Family, friends, a minister, and/or other professionals can help address these feelings.

A stigma is associated with nursing homes, such as foul odors and resident abuse and neglect. The role of the caregiver is to find a good nursing home to minimize these concerns. Caregivers should reassure their loved one that the family will ensure that his or her needs will be met in a caring and dignified manner.

Once a nursing home has been selected, take the time to review the rules, regulations, emergency/evacuation procedures, and the services provided. Know what items to provide. Acquaint yourself with the meal times, activities, and special services such as a beautician or barber. This information will help ease the transition of your loved one. Meet the staff, executive director, and the directors of the various units. Obtain advice on ensuring a smooth transition for your loved one. Determine if visiting the nursing home with your loved one is beneficial.

The move and transition can be traumatic for your loved one. Handle most of the packing and unpacking and minimize the disruption in his or her life until the move. Develop a plan for the first month. Establish a routine based on mealtimes and in-house activities. For the first week, be present as needed to help your loved one and the aides with the transition to a new routine. Review the list of weekly activities and circle those of interest. Take your loved one to the activities of interest to start the routine. Dedicate adequate time to resolve or mitigate any concerns. Focus on the positives, while working to resolve transition issues. Unless there is an important event, do not take him or her out for trips, shopping, or meals during the transition period.

One of the biggest changes may be the living quarters. Instead of a house or an apartment, your loved one only has a room or shares a room with other residents. Furnish the room in advance and make it homelike and comfortable with familiar items (pictures, bedding, etc.) Take advantage of common areas such as the lounge, dining room, patio, and foyer.

Another transition is the number of residents, visitors, and staff (care team, maintenance, etc.) in the facility at any given time. These people will add noise and activity, which in turn adds to the confusion of your loved one. Bathing arrangements may be another transition. Most nursing homes have separate bathing rooms instead of a shower in the resident's bathroom. For safety, the aides assist the residents.

The nursing home has a doctor(s) on staff for residents. Dentists and podiatrists may visit regularly. This eliminates the need for outside doctor visits but requires your loved one to adjust to new doctors. The nursing home orders and administers medication, but family members should monitor the medication plan of their loved one.

The nursing home can meet the physiological need of your loved one. Meals are served in a dining room or the resident's room if needed. Often, the nursing home has a greater role in providing the ADLs because of the cognitive and physical decline of the person. You will find a mixture of great, good, and not-as-good aides, so learn to work with all types. Develop a good relationship with the staff to make it easier to suggest ways of interacting with your loved one. Provide information to help them care for your loved one and be diligent about providing items they request. Help with your loved one's care when you can. If your loved one is unable to communicate, you may have to be present more frequently until the caregivers get to know your loved one.

Caregivers must be advocates for their loved one. Residents have a right to receive good care and be treated with dignity and respect. Random visits at different times of the day can show the staff you care about your loved one and are monitoring the care. If there are issues with your loved one's behavior, work with the staff and develop a plan to handle the issue. The staff's experience can be very valuable, and it may take a while to resolve as they try different solutions. But if your loved one is abused, not receiving proper care, or not treated with dignity and respect, take immediate action. Some aides and nurses can be rough or rude. If you repeatedly see poor treatment, begin recording the incidents with the date, staff member, and details. Discuss your concern with the staff member involved. If this does not help, have a discussion with the supervisor. Some family members have requested that certain staff members not be involved in their loved one's care. If the problem is not resolved, meet with the director of the nursing home. Another recourse is to contact a local or state long-term care ombudsman in the state Office of Aging. The mission of the ombudsman is to protect the health, safety, and rights of residents in long-term facilities. You can also file a complaint with the state's Department of Health. The goal is to try to resolve issues at the lowest level possible. Addressing poor treatment can, with time, improve the care for your loved one and other residents who have no one to speak for them. But you may feel more comfortable moving your loved one to another facility.

Nursing homes are designed to keep residents safe. They provide elevators, emergency call buttons, safety bars in the bathrooms, and the watchful eyes of staff members. But your loved one may not feel safe since he or she no longer lives at home and will want to return home. They may experience a long adjustment period.

Nursing homes help meet the social need with activities such as movies, live entertainment, and trips outside the nursing home for residents who are able. Tell family and friends about the move. Include directions and offer to bring his or her friends for a visit. Maintain contact with family and friends with cards and phone calls. Help your loved one interact with the aides, staff, roommate(s), and other residents.

Staff members can meet the esteem need for a person with Alzheimer's by treating them with dignity and respect. Family and friends, too, can help meet his or her esteem needs with regular visits and periodic gifts. A piece of jewelry, clothing, or cologne can make him or her feel special. I purchased a scarecrow from the dollar store for my mother's door, and it turned out to be one of the best dollars I have spent. She loved it. I purchased door decorations for the different seasons and holidays.

Nursing homes can meet the needs of a person with Alzheimer's in all stages of the disease. The facility keeps residents clean, fed, and safe. Social activities are provided, and in most cases residents are treated with dignity and respect. Nursing home living arrangements are not always ideal, but family members can decorate the area with familiar items and pictures.

 CHECKLIST

_____ Visit five to ten nursing homes to learn more about the care they provide.

_____ Determine if the nursing home accepts Medicaid once your loved one's money is depleted.

_____ Select two to three nursing homes that could be a fit for your loved one. Place your loved one on the waiting lists if you think a nursing home could be an option within a year.

_____ Once your loved one moves, prepare a transition plan (visits, support, etc.) for the first few months.

Chapter 23

Caregiving during Hospice Care

• • • •

I was not familiar with hospice care when my father passed away in 1987. I visited him for the Thanksgiving holiday and found he had lost more weight and was almost bedridden. My father passed away on Thanksgiving Day. Hospice could have helped support my mother in my father's final days.

Hospice is designed to provide compassionate care for a loved one and family members near the end of a person's life. The care of the person changes from treatment of a terminal illness to palliative (comfort) care. The purpose of hospice is to maximize the quality of life of the person and to support the family. Care can be in the home, care facility, or a hospice facility. A personal care plan is developed based on his or her needs and circumstances. Most hospice organizations engage a team of resources, including home health aides, nurses, doctors, social workers, chaplains, and volunteers. Hospice provides some medications and supplies, help with ADLs, light housekeeping, pain management, emotional support, preparing the person and family for death with dignity, and bereavement counseling.[1]

Typically, families wait too late to engage hospice and do not receive the full benefit of this service. Work with your family doctor and start contacting hospice to learn about the offering. Speak with others with hospice experience to gain valuable insight. Selecting a hospice agency before it is needed will make this time less difficult. Hospice services are covered by Medicare, Medicaid, and most insurance companies.

My brothers and I did not want to wait too late to take full advantage of hospice so we began investigating agencies early. We had heard that some persons with Alzheimer's were in hospice care for multiple years.

To: Mike, Ron   Date: 3/9/11
From: Carol   Subject: Hospice
I did some hospice research on the web last night. I saw nothing where it increased the expected eligibility lifetime of the person with Alzheimer's above six months. Some of the data showed Alzheimer's patients are in hospice on average 8.6 months. The information suggests putting the person in hospice when they are in the final stages of the disease. Mom is probably at the end of the middle stage.

To: Carol, Ron   Date: 3/11/11
From: Mike   Subject: Re: Hospice
I agree. Mom is probably at the end of the middle stage.

On page 4 of the book I emailed earlier, it states a person can receive Medicare hospice benefits when all of the following conditions are met:

- You're eligible for Medicare Part A (hospital insurance).
- Your doctor and the hospice medical director certify that you're terminally ill and have six months or less to live if your illness runs its normal course.

- You sign a statement choosing hospice care instead of other Medicare-covered benefits to treat your terminal illness.
- You get care from a Medicare-approved hospice program.[2]

Alzheimer's patients could be getting around this by: (1) using the fact that a person with Alzheimer's has a terminal illness and (2) declaring early that the person has six months or less to live because medically it may be more difficult to estimate the day of death for an Alzheimer's patient than, say, for a cancer patient.

Maybe sometime when I am in Wilmington this year I will set up appointments with hospice providers to talk generically about the process (that is, timeline, paperwork, benefits, costs, care, etc.) for getting the service implemented. This way we will already know the process and have a contact if we need to move in that way.

My brothers and I began exploring hospice services and benefits in 2011. We did our research and spoke with two hospice providers. We were mainly concerned about the management of our mother's care. Hospice focuses on comfort versus treatment. We wanted our family, with input from her doctor, making decisions regarding her care. I spoke with family members of residents utilizing hospice and received these tips:

- Select an agency that provides care seven days a week since a person may pass away on a weekend.
- Change agencies if the care is not satisfactory.
- Hospice care can last more than six months. One loved one was in hospice almost two years. A re-evaluation was required every ninety days, but hospice completed the required paperwork.
- Hospice provided a lot of useful end-of-life information.
- The hospice visits can increase as the need increases.

- Their loved one actually received more care because the residential facility continued providing the same level of care.
- Their loved one was never denied any care, treatment, or payment their loved one needed.

To: Mike, Carol   Date: 9/28/11

From: Ron   Subject: Hospice Care

After review of the hospice information, I do not think Mom qualifies for that move. I base my decision on the following assumptions:

- Most patients would be bedridden.
- Her current care and hospital care are very good.
- Mom is still mobile and gets around. Her facility provides that type of environment.

Mom is a fighter. In my opinion, hospice care is a concession. And she's just not ready to concede.

From what I have gathered from your reports of Mom's lung and coughing condition, it has not been deemed terminal, but treatable. Hospice is inevitable. But I just don't think it's now.

Just my thoughts.

My brothers and I decided not to pursue hospice at that time. Since we had done the research, it was easy to revisit our decision on a regular basis. Indirectly we were evaluating her cognitive capability, physical ability, and quality of life. We revisited hospice care when she stopped eating a week before she passed away.

To: Mike   Date: 6/8/14

From: Carol   Subject: Hospice

We may want to consider hospice. Let's wait until after your visit to even bring it up. I wouldn't be surprised if her facility brings it up again...maybe as we get closer.

Right now Mom has the sniffles. Maybe it's from allergies because she wasn't put back on allergy medicine when she returned from the hospital. She was outside yesterday which I want them to continue. So if something happens where Mom needs more than her facility can provide, do we send her to the hospital or let hospice handle...whatever that means. I really would prefer Mom to pass away at her home instead of a hospital.

My mother essentially stopped eating, and her condition continued to deteriorate.

To: Carol   Date: 6/10/14

From: Mike   Subject: Next Steps

I would do the following this evening:

1. Contact hospice and tell them you want Mom under their care at her facility ASAP.
2. Inform her doctor of these plans.
3. Inform your pastor of these plans.

Pre-planning for funeral arrangements can be done earlier in the journey. Pre-planning allows families to think about an appropriate and meaningful memorial during a less stressful time. Mike and I did not pre-plan but made key decisions such as the number and location of funeral services, cemetery, and homegoing celebration program. One of the more pressing issues was my mother's burial attire. As she lost weight toward the end of her life, her dress size changed so we had to select and purchase a new dress. Also, we decided at the last minute to place a hat in the casket for the Cleveland funeral service, since Mom always said, "A woman isn't dressed unless she has a hat."

End-of-life care is difficult because it is near the end. The hospice staff can keep the loved one free of pain and comfortable in a soothing environment. The hospice staff can prepare families for the end. At the end, what really counts is the life the person has lived, the love from the lives the person has touched, and his or her eternal life.

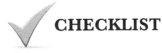 **CHECKLIST**

_____ Become familiar with local hospice agencies.
_____ Talk to others about their experiences with hospice.
_____ Consider pre-need arrangements with a funeral home.

Part VI

Advice for the Caregiver

Chapter 24

Mind the Gap

• • • •

It did not take long to realize it was difficult to meet all of my mother's needs, all of the time. In many instances, I was trying to balance my personal needs with Mom's needs. Sometimes as I was leaving her facility I would sense she wanted me to remain longer. Many times I remained until she was in a better frame of mind. Sometimes I had to leave. Mom was usually fine if I was going to work or church. But a few times she let me know I was making other things more important than her. Whether she said something or not, I often felt guilty leaving her at her memory care facility.

The Caregiving Principle™, introduced in chapter 4, is the basis for this book. It states:

Needs of the Person – Needs Filled by the Person = Needs to Be Filled by the Caregiver(s).

The principle provides a simple framework for understanding a person with Alzheimer's. If taken literally, caregivers will have to fill all of a loved one's needs that he or she cannot fill all of the time. But healthy people do not always meet their needs. They may have a need for a social activity but instead remain at work to finish a report. They may be hungry but decide to finish the report to arrive home earlier. Similarly, it is difficult to meet all of a loved one's needs all of the time. The role of the caregiver is to "mind the gap." "Mind the gap" is a United Kingdom term for rail passengers to watch for the gap between the train door and the station platform. In essence, the same is true for caregivers. Caregivers must anticipate, understand, watch out for, and minimize the impact of these caregiving gaps on their loved one. It is critical that caregivers "mind the gap."

Physiological Need Gaps

Physiological need gaps may be difficult to determine because a loved one may be unable to communicate or remember he or she is hungry, thirsty, tired, or have to use the restroom.

When our mother's behavior was different, I wondered if she had slept well the night before. The night staff kept records, but if Mom did not get up or if she was asleep when they checked on her they may not have known she had a restless night. Sometimes I continued the investigation with my brothers.

To: Ron, Mike   Date: 9/20/06
From: Carol   Subject: Mom having an off day
Give Mom a call. She's having an "off day," as she calls it. Mike, did she seem unusually disoriented last night when she called you, or did it appear she was up late?

To: Carol, Ron   Date: 9/20/06
From: Mike   Subject: Re: Mom having an off day

No more disoriented last night than in the last one to two weeks. She didn't call after 10 p.m. She called tonight a few times.

In this instance, our mother gave no indication she was up late or unusually troubled the night before.

Caregivers may not always be aware of gaps. For example, my mother's primary care physician observed her walking and noticed her gait was not quite right. He recommended physical therapy. I did not notice the change and appreciated her doctor identifying the gap.

Sometimes Mom's medical appointment may have run late. To manage this gap, I kept snacks and water in the car, and the staff at her facility saved her meal for her return.

My brothers and I managed some of our mother's IADLs, and these were usually the items that temporarily fell in the gap. For instance, I made sure she had medication, even if we could not resolve which insurance should pay for the medication until a month later.

Safety Need Gaps

Gaps in physical safety can occur when caregivers assume their loved one needs less supervision than he or she actually needs. Chapter 19, I Never Thought She Would... describes the incident that was a huge safety gap. The incident put Mom in harm's way, increased her anxiety, and reduced her retirement funds.

At times I chose to leave Mom alone in a medical building lobby while I parked the car. This was a gap I purposely managed because I believed if she wandered away she would not get far. I was thankful she never wandered away.

Hospitalizations decreased Mom's sense of security, but I could not be with her a hundred percent of the time. I was with her in the emergency room until she was admitted to meet her nursing team. I visited Mom before work, during my lunchtime, and then in the evening to meet with her doctor. Alvin and Mike also visited to minimize the impact of this gap.

Social Need Gaps

Mom and I had gaps in our interaction while I was traveling. I gave her and the staff advance notice, and I sent a postcard. Ron and Mike called more often.

Our mother's phone communication with her relatives fell in the gap. As the disease progressed, she had less of a desire to speak to relatives. Sometimes these calls reminded her of how much she could not remember. Mom also started having difficulty maintaining conversations. I should have called and spoken to family members on the speakerphone. Maybe she would have spoken; but at a minimum she would have heard the familiar voice of a close relative.

Self-Esteem Gaps

Hospitalizations sometimes created self-esteem gaps because I focused on improving my mother's health so she could return to the familiarity of her memory care facility. Sometimes I was firmer with Mom than I wanted to be to get her to do physical therapy or to eat. I always told Mom I would not ask her to do what she could not do. In the end, I could not force her to do something she did not want to do.

Caregivers must meet the needs loved ones cannot provide for themselves. Caregivers should identify situations where gaps in meeting the needs could occur. Develop a plan to avoid or manage these gaps in care.

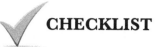 **CHECKLIST**

_____ List the potential physiological, safety, social, and self-esteem gaps for your loved one.

_____ Develop a plan to avoid or manage these gaps.

_____ Evaluate and adjust the plan as necessary.

Chapter 25

What about Me?

• • • •

In the fall, as the daylight faded, my mother rushed me out of her room so I did not have to drive home in the dark. She said, "I want you to arrive home safely because I'd be lost without you." I worried about being able to care for Mom. A car accident or a normal illness could have prevented me from providing care. Caregiving was a balancing act between my needs and my mother's. If I did not take care of myself I would be unable to care for her.

A good friend shared a song lyric with me that directly addresses caregivers. It is "The leaning tree is not always the first to fall."[1] It was her reminder that I must take care of myself. I knew caregiving could affect my physical, mental, and spiritual health. I was aware of the caregiver stress symptoms and fortunately only had them for a short period. The symptoms are:

1. Denial about the disease and its effect on the person who's been diagnosed.
2. Anger at the person with Alzheimer's or others, anger that no cure exists, or anger that people don't understand what's going on.

3. Social withdrawal from friends and activities that once brought pleasure.
4. Anxiety about facing another day and what the future holds.
5. Depression that begins to break your spirit and affect your ability to cope.
6. Exhaustion that makes it nearly impossible to complete necessary daily tasks.
7. Sleeplessness caused by a never-ending list of concerns.
8. Irritability that leads to moodiness and triggers negative responses and actions.
9. Lack of concentration that makes it difficult to perform familiar tasks.
10. Health problems that begin to take their toll, both mentally and physically.[2]

The Alzheimer's Association reports some startling statistics:

- "Approximately 30 percent to 40 percent of family caregivers of people with dementia suffer from depression, compared with 5 to 17 percent of non-caregivers of similar ages."[3]
- "Family and other unpaid caregivers of people with Alzheimer's or other dementia are more likely than non-caregivers to have high levels of stress hormones, reduced immune function, slow wound healing, new hypertension and new coronary heart disease."[4]
- "Most family caregivers report 'a good amount' to 'a great deal' of caregiving strain concerning financial issues (47 percent) and family relationships (52 percent)."[5]

These statistics are not intended to scare caregivers, but rather to raise awareness of the difficult task ahead. Avoid becoming a statistic. As a caregiver, I always felt I should do more. Another task would come up, but I could not do it all. I focused on Mom's physiological and safety needs and tried not to feel guilty when I could not meet other needs. I had to take care of myself so I could continue to take care of my mother. Caregivers can apply Maslow's Hierarchy of Needs to themselves to ensure they are taking care of themselves and are managing any gaps.

To manage the caregiving stress:

- I maintained a strong relationship with God and my church family, realizing God was in control.
- I maintained a strong relationship with Alvin, family, and friends. My circle of support was in an ideal position to identify and address caregiving stress. I also had to understand the impact of my caregiving on them.
- I shared caregiving responsibilities with my brothers when possible.
- Alvin and I took at least two vacations every year. Mike became the primary contact for Mom's needs while we were away.
- I set aside at least two vacation days a year just for me. Called my sanity days, I usually took four half-days of vacation to sleep in, go to the beautician, or take a tennis lesson.
- I managed my health with the same rigor as I did for Mom.
- The family members of the other memory care residents were my support group. We shared stories and encouraged each other.
- I sometimes included my personal feelings in my emails to my brothers, which was therapeutic. Some caregivers keep a journal.
- I reduced stress from other aspects of my life. For instance, often I commuted by bus to avoid stressful rush-hour driving.

Some caregivers add to their stress by wondering, Will I develop Alzheimer's? Everyone contemplates this topic as they age and start to misplace items or lose their train of thought. Is it a "senior moment" or the early stages of Alzheimer's disease? I've included no emails on this subject because my brothers and I never discussed it in person, by phone, or through emails. The chance of developing the disease increases with age, and my family has been blessed with longevity. A person with a family history of Alzheimer's may have a risk gene that increases the likelihood of developing the disease.[6] Some people with a family history of Alzheimer's will undergo genetic testing to determine if they have an increased risk. I have not chosen to be tested although my mother, an immediate family member, had Alzheimer's disease. So what about me?

I choose to focus my energy on activities that promote a healthy lifestyle.

- I visit my doctor(s) regularly and have an annual physical. Many risk factors for heart disease such as high blood pressure, high cholesterol, diabetes, being overweight, and lack of exercise are bad for your brain.[7]
- I drink plenty of water, and I am working on improving my eating habits.
- I exercise regularly, playing tennis and working out in the gym.
- I get plenty of rest most nights. I try to make sleep a priority. Persons who snore or feel tired after a good amount of sleep should be evaluated for sleep apnea, a risk factor for Alzheimer's.[8]
- I remain socially involved with church, cultural, and alumni activities and travel. Many of the activities that met my mother's social need also met mine.
- I exercise my mind. I am open to trying and learning new things. I have fallen in love with Sudoku puzzles. In writing this book, I have learned about writing and the publishing industry.

- I minimize stress by focusing on things I can control. Items I cannot control cause unnecessary anxiety and waste time and energy I can devote to more productive matters. I know God is in control.
- I keep abreast of new developments in the prevention and reversal of Alzheimer's disease.
- I support my local Alzheimer's Association so we can end the disease. I am an advocate and have supported the fundraisers, including the Walk to End Alzheimer's as a participant and volunteer.

Although Alzheimer's is prevalent in my family, I do not dwell on my likelihood of developing this disease. Instead I rely on my faith in God. Mom was an example of how to live with Alzheimer's with grace, dignity, and humor. She learned to be content in her situation. Sometimes Mom said, "I'm doing well. I like living here. The people are nice. I'm not in pain. I wake up every morning and thank God for keeping me. I do the same before going to bed. God's grace is sufficient for me."

Caregivers should make a conscious effort to reduce stress in their lives by obtaining additional help and taking regular breaks (respite care) from caregiving. Taking time for rejuvenation can reduce stress and provide a healthier outlook on the entire situation.

 CHECKLIST

_____ Recognize the signs of caregiver stress.

_____ Make a personal assessment of the impact of caregiving. Identify two things to change to reduce the stress of caregiving.

_____ Schedule regular doctor visits and remain current on medical screenings.

Chapter 26

Keep It Simple

• • • •

Managing my mother's care was time consuming and sometimes stressful. I worked full-time and had obligations to my family, church, and other organizations. I had to identify ways to simplify my responsibilities to avoid becoming overwhelmed.

The caregiving role is extremely challenging, but I felt I was a good and consistent caregiver throughout this journey. Here are some examples of how I simplified my role.

- In memory care, initially, I scheduled Mom's medical appointments around 9 a.m. When I informed her in advance, she called incessantly the night before to clarify the details. I began leaving a typewritten note the day before with appointment details, but she still called. Then I started scheduling Mom's appointments mid-morning or afternoon so she could maintain her waking, dressing, and eating routine.
- When selecting doctors for less critical medical issues, proximity to Mom's facility and availability of Friday appointments (for Mike to accompany her) became considerations.

- I shifted many of my errands (shopping mall, shoe repair, etc.) to the area near Mom's memory care facility to minimize travel time.

- Alvin and I had scheduled a Thanksgiving vacation before Mom's move to Delaware. I felt guilty leaving Mom during Thanksgiving week to vacation, but I went. I learned that holiday celebrations are important, but the celebration does not have to occur on the actual day. Her facility prepared a great noontime holiday meal followed by relevant festivities throughout the day. Therefore, some holiday celebrations were early or delayed. Mom enjoyed the celebrations whenever they occurred.

- My mother never returned (alive) to Cleveland after moving to Delaware. The long trip, by car or plane, would have been difficult for everyone involved. I ensured Mom saw family and friends whenever they were anywhere near Delaware. She met with a busload of her Cleveland church family at a Delaware shopping mall, and Mike and I took Mom to her niece's wedding in Maryland. I drove two of her Cleveland sisters, who were on a church trip, from Baltimore to Wilmington to visit Mom. She enjoyed every opportunity to fellowship with family and friends.

- Each year brought a change in the Medicare and insurance company's drug formulary. This impacted which insurance (Medicare, pharmacy, private medical) covered Mom's inhaler medications. After a few hectic Januarys, I began to accumulate (refilled the prescription at the earliest date) enough medication in the later part of the year to cover Mom's needs in January while insurance coverage was resolved.

- When our mother was scheduled for a surgery, Mike hired a private caregiver to prevent her from eating or drinking before the procedure. We were able to get a good night's sleep before what would most likely be a hectic day.

- In multiple instances Mike and I felt a particular company owed our mother money because of a mistake with billing or insurance coverage. We knew it could be a challenge (time, stress, waiting on hold, and aggravation) recovering the money. If the amount Mom was owed was below a threshold amount, we would not pursue.

Caregivers can explore how to simplify their lives with such things as automated bill pay, freezing meals, having a neighborhood teenager help with yard work, or even using professionals for routine or non-routine services such as window washing, mulching, or painting. Keeping caregiving simple can save money, reduce aggravation, make caregiving less stressful, and free up time for more rewarding activities.

 CHECKLIST

_____ Join an Alzheimer's Association support group to learn how to simplify caregiving.

_____ Peruse the Alzheimer's Association website to investigate ways of simplifying or sharing your caregiving responsibilities.

Chapter 27

Be Grateful for God's Rays of Hope

• • • •

My family experienced a great deal during our mother's eleven-year battle with Alzheimer's disease. Our faith in God and each other sustained us and gave us hope. Often, my brothers and I paused and expressed gratitude to God and each other for our progress on this journey.

This was a difficult eleven-year journey, but God was with us from the beginning. It started when my brothers and I discovered Mom had memory issues and sought out medical care. We witnessed her on-going confusion, delusions, and mistrust of us. We moved her from her home of twenty years to assisted living when she became the target of a scam. She could have been seriously harmed or killed, but God spared her life. The next year we uprooted her from Cleveland to a secure memory care facility near my home.

Throughout the journey God blessed us with rays of hope. Mike was very good at reminding us how far we had come and how much we should be grateful for, and we all became better at showing our gratitude.

It was a blessing to reflect and thank God for our progress and remain hopeful not knowing what was ahead. Here are a few examples.

To: Ron, Mike   Date: 9/30/03
From: Carol   Subject: Good Morning

I took a half-day of vacation to get a little extra sleep and get caught up on personal things. So, as I get up this morning, I am thankful to God for all He has done for me and my family. But most of all I am thankful and blessed to have two brothers like you. We (with the help of God) accomplished a great deal this past week. But what I'm grateful for is how we accomplished our goal. We worked together, came up with ideas, and upgraded the idea to the best solution. And we did it all working with Mom in a compassionate way. So as I thank God for this beautiful Tuesday morning, I also thank Him for blessing me with brothers like you.

To: Carol, Mike   Date: 10/1/03
From: Ron   Subject: No subject

This past week was great!!!!!!!! We got to spend some time together and got an awful lot accomplished. I left Cleveland very satisfied and happy.

I've read your emails, and I see you left Cleveland feeling the same way I did. Everything went so well!!!!

I can't believe we got so much done including the extra items we found along the way. I'm still amazed.

To: Ron, Mike Date: 12/16/03

From: Carol Subject: Dec 13-15 Trip Report

Attached are my updates. Here are three general observations:

- Memory is still a problem, but she seems less agitated about the situation.
- House seemed to be very orderly, not as much paper clutter.
- Mom is more receptive to anything we recommend. She is extremely grateful to all of us for our support and patience.

To: Carol, Ron Date: 1/17/05

From: Mike Subject: Re: Jan 14-16 Trip Report

Great trip!! Thanks for making this happen.

Mom's memory issue, which can be disheartening at times, especially when you are there experiencing it, probably has not worsened over the last few months. Assisted living is working out, and Mom is making the transition. CRITICAL assisted living issues have subsided, and there have been no issues with BANKS! There is nothing urgently critical (safety, health, finances, etc.) we are dealing with in regard to Mom, which is a blessing. This is really a good time.

Life is not easy for Mom, but she bravely continues to look forward to each day. We need to continue what we are doing (telephone calls, mail, visits, etc.) letting her know how much we love and appreciate her for what she has done and is doing.

To: Carol, Ron   Date: 2/11/06
From: Mike   Subject: Re: MAKING THINGS UP

There are several blessings we sometimes overlook since Mom moved to Delaware:

- Mom does not feel the need to have a key for her room and to lock her outside door.
- Mom lets the caregivers launder her clothing and linens.
- She lets the caregivers assist her with getting a shower two to three times per week.
- She hasn't complained about not being in the assisted living part of the building even though she passes through it at least once a week.
- As far as we know Mom has not recently tried to leave the memory care facility, one of the biggest reasons we moved her out of assisted living.
- Her health has remained good. Her replaced knee has not been a problem.
- She gets to go to church regularly.
- Carol gets to see and check up on any issues regularly.
- No one has to travel to Mom's location to get her to non-routine medical appointments.
- Mom reached her eighty-sixth birthday.
- Mom enjoys where she is living.
- Mom is safe and is getting good care.

Let's count our blessings. Name them one by one. There are more so add them to the list. Any one of these items could have been a major issue. Things that have come up like the telephone charges do not reach the status of being an issue.

To: Mike   Date: 8/10/13

From: Carol   Subject: Count Your Blessings

Thanks so much for coming to Delaware to be with Mom. It's sort of amazing how a lot of things are going well:

- Mom lost some unneeded weight.
- Mom is doing well on less medicine (less cost and probably less confusion).
- She is probably mentally and physically close to her pre-hospitalization mental and physical state—you may be a better judge of this.
- She has things like the hospital bed per her lung doctor's recommendation and has new special shoes that may help her walk better.

As you say. Count your blessings. Count them one by one.

My gratitude to God is overflowing. I am grateful that Elizabeth T. Boyd was my mother. I am grateful my brothers and I, with medical and caregiving professionals, were able to provide excellent care for her. I am grateful she moved to Delaware and eventually considered her memory care facility her family and her home. I am grateful for the love and care her new family provided. I am grateful for my family, my friends, and her friends who supported us along the way. I am grateful for all the precious memories Mom and I created together. I am grateful for the life lessons she instilled in me such as faith, honesty, and achievement. I am grateful my mother passed away peacefully with family in the comfort of her room. I am grateful for the legacy she left that will live on through her family and the lives of the people she touched. I am grateful for the peace that only God can give.

Our mother, Elizabeth T. Boyd, went home to be with God June 15, 2014. This journey was Mom's journey, and she approached it bravely with dignity, grace, and humor. I was comforted because I felt Mom decided it was time to pass on. She lived her ninety-four years of life preparing to transition to a better place. She was ready to go home to be with our Lord. Our family was there for her. We told her we loved her, and we thanked her for being our mom. We prayed with her. Gospel music played in her room, and the caregivers periodically played her Mother's Day music box with the hymn "Amazing Grace." The cause of death on her death certificate was Alzheimer Dementia. Following a viewing in Delaware, her body returned to Cleveland for a funeral and burial.

Thank you, caregivers, for reading this book and for all you are doing for your loved one. My prayer is that *H.O.P.E. for the Alzheimer's Journey* will bless and encourage you and help you to have a less stressful and more rewarding experience as a caregiver. May God give you and your family rays of hope, strength, love, and encouragement to continue your Alzheimer's journey.

 CHECKLIST

_____ Be grateful for your progress along the journey.

_____ Take time to thank those who help you. Take time to thank yourself.

_____ Draw upon past successes for hope and strength for the remainder of the journey.

Appendix 1

The Global Deterioration Scale (GDS)

• • • •

(Choose the most appropriate global stage based upon cognition and function, and CHECK ONLY ONE)

1. **No subjective complaints of memory deficit.** No memory deficit evident on clinical interview.

2. **Subjective complaints of memory deficit**, most frequently in following areas:

    a) forgetting where one has placed familiar objects;

    b) forgetting names one formerly knew well.

    No objective evidence of memory deficit on clinical interview.

    No objective deficit in employment or social situations.

    Appropriate concern with respect to symptomatology.

3. **Earliest clear-cut deficits.**

    Manifestations in more than one of the following areas:

    a) patient may have gotten lost when traveling to an unfamiliar location.

    b) co-workers become aware of patient's relatively poor performance.

c) word and/or name finding deficit become evident to intimates.

d) patient may read a passage or book and retain relatively little material.

e) patient may demonstrate decreased facility remembering names upon introduction to new people.

f) patient may have lost or misplaced an object of value.

g) concentration deficit may be evident on clinical testing.

Objective evidence of memory deficit obtained **only with an intensive interview**.

Decreased performance in demanding employment and social settings.

Denial begins to become manifest in patient.

Mild to moderate anxiety frequently accompanies symptoms.

4. **Clear-cut deficit on careful clinical interview.**

Deficit manifest in following areas:

a) decreased knowledge of current and recent events.

b) may exhibit some deficit in memory of one's personal history.

c) concentration deficit elicited on serial subtractions.

d) decreased ability to travel, **handle finances**, etc.

Frequently no deficit in following areas:

a) orientation to time and place.

b) recognition of familiar persons and faces.

c) ability to travel to familiar locations.

Inability to perform complex tasks.

Denial is dominant defense mechanism.

Flattening of affect and withdrawal from challenging situations.

5. **Patient can no longer survive without some assistance.**

Patient is unable during interview to recall a major relevant aspect of their current life, for example:

a) their address or telephone number of many years.

b) the names of close members of their family (such as grandchildren).

c) the name of the high school or college from which they graduated.

Frequently some disorientation to time (date, day of the week, season, etc.) or to place.

An educated person may have difficulty counting back from forty by fours or from twenty by twos.

Persons at this stage retain knowledge of many major facts regarding themselves and others.

They invariably know their own names and generally know their spouse's and children's names.

They require no assistance with toileting or eating, but may have difficulty choosing the proper clothing to wear.

6. May occasionally forget the name of the spouse upon whom they are entirely dependent for survival.

Will be **largely unaware of all recent events and experiences in their lives.**

Retain some knowledge of their surroundings; the year, the season, etc.

May have difficulty counting by ones from ten, both backward and sometimes forward.

Will require some assistance with activities of daily living:

a) may become incontinent.

b) will require travel assistance but occasionally will be able to travel to familiar locations.

Diurnal rhythm frequently disturbed.

Almost always recall their own name.

Frequently continue to be able to distinguish familiar from unfamiliar persons in their environment.

Personality and emotional changes occur. These are quite variable and include:

a) delusional behavior: for example, patients may accuse their spouse of being an imposter; may talk to imaginary figures in the environment, or to their own reflection in the mirror.

b) obsessive symptoms, for example, person may continually repeat simple cleaning activities.

c) anxiety symptoms, agitation, and even previously non-existent violent behavior may occur.

d) cognitive abulia, that is, loss of willpower because an individual cannot carry a thought long enough to determine a purposeful course of action.

7. **All verbal abilities are lost over the course of this stage.**
Early in this stage words and phrases are spoken, but speech is very circumscribed.

Later there is no serviceable speech at all—only unintelligible utterances with rare emergence of seemingly forgotten words and phrases.

Incontinent; requires assistance toileting and feeding.

Basic psychomotor skills (for example, ability to walk) **are lost with the progression of this stage.**

The brain appears to no longer be able to tell the body what to do. Generalized rigidity and developmental neurologic reflexes are frequently present.

Reisberg, B., Ferris, S.H., de Leon, M.J., et. al., The global deterioration scale for assessment of primary degenerative dementia. *American Journal of Psychiatry*, 1982, 139:1136-1139.

Appendix 2

Summary of Book Resources

• • • •

Books, Pamphlets. Reports, and Training

- Coste, Joanne Koenig and Robert Butler, *Learning to Speak Alzheimer's: A Groundbreaking Approach for Everyone Dealing with the Disease*, New York: Mariner Books, 2004.
- Mace, Nancy L. and Peter V. Rabins, *The 36-Hour Day: A Family Guide to Caring for People Who Have Alzheimer's Disease, Related Dementias, and Memory Loss*, Baltimore: Johns Hopkins University Press, 2017.
- Morris, Virginia, *How to Care for Aging Parents: A Complete Guide*, New York: Workman Publishing Company, 1996.
- The Alzheimer's Association, *2017 Alzheimer's Disease Facts and Figures*, Alzheimers Dement 2017; 13:325-373, https://www.alz.org/documents_custom/2017-facts-and-figures.pdf.
- The Alzheimer's Association, "Communication, Tips for Successful Communication during All Stages of Alzheimer's Disease," rev. May 2017, 770-10-0018, http://www.alz.org/national/documents/brochure_communication.pdf.
- The Alzheimer's Association, essentiALZ˚, online dementia training from the Alzheimer's Association and HealthCare Interactive Inc., http://www.alz.org/essentialz/.

- The Alzheimer's Association, "Personal Care: Assisting a Person with Middle- or Late-Stage Dementia with Daily Needs," rev. Dec. 2016, 770-10-00191, https://www.alz.org/national/documents/brochure_personalcare.pdf.
- The Alzheimer's Association, "Staying Safe: Steps to Take for a Person with Dementia," rev. Dec. 2016, 775-10-0014, https://www.alz.org/national/documents/brochure_stayingsafe.pdf.
- *The Bible*—King James Version.
- U. S. Department of Health and Human Services, NIH National Institute on Aging, "Home Safety and Alzheimer's Disease," updated July 25, 2017, https://www.nia.nih.gov/health/home-safety-and-alzheimers-disease.

Businesses, Government, and Organizations

- AARP, Caregiving, www.AARP.org.
- Alzheimer's Disease Research Centers, https://www.nia.nih.gov/health/alzheimers-disease-research-centers#nacc.
- Genworth Financial, Inc., "Compare Long-Term Care Costs across the United States," https://www.genworth.com/corporate/about-genworth/industry-expertise/cost-of-care.html.
- Medicaid, https://www.medicaid.gov.
- Medicare.gov, https://www.medicare.gov.
- Medicare.gov, Nursing Home Comparison, https://www.medicare.gov/nursinghomecompare/search.html.
- The Alzheimer's Association, (www.alz.org).
- The Alzheimer's Association 24/7 Helpline – 1-800-272-3900.
- The Alzheimer's Association, "MedicAlert + Alzheimer's Association Safe Return, http://www.alz.org/care/dementia-medic-alert-safe-return.asp.

- The Alzheimer's Disease Education and Referral Center (ADEAR), National Institutes of Health (NIH), National Institute on Aging (NIA), www.nia.nih.gov/alzheimers.
- The Alzheimer's Store, www.alzstore.com.
- *U.S. News and World Report,* Nursing Homes Ratings, http://health.usnews.com/best-nursing-homes.

ACKNOWLEDGMENTS

All praise and glory to my God who inspired me to write this book and opened doors for publication. May this book bless and encourage caregivers and those persons suffering with Alzheimer's disease.

I am grateful to David Hancock and Terry Whalin of Morgan James Publishing who believed in my book but, more important, believed in me. Also thanks to my publishing and marketing team, Bonnie Rauch, Jim Howard, Nickcole Watkins, and the entire Morgan James family.

Thanks to all of my family. A special thanks goes to my husband, Alvin, the love of my life. Alvin has shared his love, understanding, and unending support of me, especially throughout this project. My brother, Mike, has been part of this project from the beginning, providing early feedback on content and organization to the very end. My sister-in-law, Judy, provided early feedback and encouragement at just the right times. To my niece, Moriah, whom I have watched grow into a fun, loving, and responsible woman. And to my late brother, Ron, who provided early feedback on this project. I still miss him. Thanks to my extended family for a lifetime of support and to my church family, Canaan Baptist Church, for their love, spiritual support, and my continued spiritual development.

The early readers of my book provided their precious time to review and give invaluable feedback. They helped me make a step-change improvement. Thank you to Lauren Anderson, Judith C. Boyd, Michael G. Boyd, Debbie Bullock, Ed.D., Wendy Hicks-Powers, and

Lisa Horton, MD. Thanks to Mary Busha, Your Time to Write! for early edits of the book and The Editorial Attic for final editing. Also thanks to Tawny Johnson, D. C. Jacobson & Associates, for useful feedback on the book proposal, title, and manuscript.

I have grown as an author with the help of:

- Marlene Bagnull, Director and my instructors and network from the Greater Philadelphia Christian Writers Conference including Dr. Harold L. Arnold Jr. who encouraged me to "dive in."
- My instructors and network from the Writer's Digest Conference and multiple Writer's Digest online courses.
- Mentorship from Mary Busha, Kelly Wilson, Jacki Kelly, and Lauren Anderson.

A sincere thanks to Dr. Barry Reisberg for granting me permission to include The Global Deterioration Scale (GDS) in my book. A special thanks to the Alzheimer's Association for granting me permission to use information from their website.

Finally, a very special thanks to family, friends, caregivers, strangers, and medical professionals who supported my mother and family during our Alzheimer's journey. I am especially grateful to her care teams at her assisted-living and memory care facilities. Words cannot express the depth of gratitude I have for all of you.

To God Be the Glory!

DEAR CAREGIVER

Thank you for reading my book. Please stay in contact by providing comments and feedback on the book at Carolbamos.com. There you can download some of the tools and sign up for my newsletter. You can follow me on Facebook and Twitter or write about H.O.P.E. on social media. Please consider leaving a review on Amazon, Barnes and Noble, or Goodreads. You can also be a blessing to others by providing this book to a friend or family member who is caring for someone with Alzheimer's disease.

I pray that my book has **H**elped you to become **O**rganized and **P**repared with **E**ducation, tools, advice, and encouragement to be a good caregiver to your loved one. Continue to enjoy your loved one and let him or her know you are there for love and support. Please reach out to family, friends, medical professionals and the Alzheimer's Association for help. Also reach out to God for continued strength, wisdom, and encouragement. May God continue to send you rays of hope for the rest of your journey.

God Bless You,
Carol B. Amos

*****

To schedule seminars or workshops or for bulk sales, please visit my website at Carolbamos.com.

ABOUT THE AUTHOR

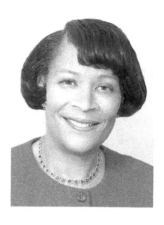

Carol B. Amos started her Alzheimer's journey when her mother started having memory problems. Carol has immersed herself in Alzheimer's education by reading and attending conferences, workshops, and support groups. Carol is a CARES Dementia Specialist and is Alzheimer's Association essentiALZ Plus certified. She was the winner of the 2012 "Your Favorite Memory" essay contest sponsored by the Delaware Valley Alzheimer's Association. She has a passion to share her knowledge and make the journey for Alzheimer's caregivers less stressful and more rewarding. She is also working to help eliminate Alzheimer's disease as an Alzheimer's Association volunteer, fundraiser, and advocate.

Carol has a B.S. and M.Eng. in chemical engineering from Cornell University. She retired from a thirty-five-year career at The DuPont Company. She is active in her church (youth ministry, women's ministry, usher board, and construction committee). She has been married to her husband, Alvin, for nineteen years. She enjoys tennis, travel, and gardening at her home in Delaware.

END NOTES

Introduction

1. *2007 Alzheimer's Disease Facts and Figures*, The Alzheimer's Association, page 17, https://www.alz.org/national/documents/Report_2007FactsAndFigures.pdf.

2. *2017 Alzheimer's Disease Facts and Figures*, The Alzhcimer's Association, pages 6-7, https://www.alz.org/documents_custom/2017-facts-and-figures.pdf.

Chapter 1

1. Ibid., pages 18 and 33.

Chapter 2

1. Ibid., page 40.

Chapter 3

1. Ibid., page 6.

2. Peter V. Rabins, MD, MPH, *Memory: Your Personal Guide to Alzheimer's Disease and Dementia*, The Johns Hopkins White Papers, Johns Hopkins Medicine, 2012 Remedy Health Media, LLC, pages 38-39.

3. "Know the 10 Signs," *The Alzheimer's Association*, 2017, http://www.alz.org/national/documents/checklist_10signs.pdf.

4. "Signs and Symptoms," Cognitive Neurology and Alzheimer's Disease Center, Northwestern Medicine, Northwestern

University, Feinberg School of Medicine, http://www.brain. northwestern.edu/dementia/ad/signs.html.

5. Ricardo S. Osorio, MD, et al, "Sleep-Disordered Breathing Advances Cognitive Decline in the Elderly," *Neurology* (April 15, 2015).

6. Peter V. Rabins, MD, MPH, *Memory: Your Personal Guide to Alzheimer's Disease*, page 46.

7. Alzheimer's Disease Research Centers, National Institute on Aging, https://www.nia.nih.gov/health/alzheimers-disease-research-centers#nacc.

8. Specific Internet source unknown.

9. Barbara Bridges, RN, MSN, MSHCHM, MBA, "Handling Memory Loss," WebMD, 2003.

10. Specific Internet source unknown.

11. Virginia Morris, *How to Care for Aging Parents: A Complete Guide* (New York: Workman Publishing Company, 1996).

Chapter 4

1. Enid Kassner, AARP Public Policy Institute, and Beth Jackson, The MEDSTAT Group "Determining Comparable Levels of Functional Disability," *AARP*, April 1, 1998, http://www.aarp. org/home-garden/livable-communities/info-1998/aresearch-import-710-IB32.html.

2. Neel Burton, MD, "Our Hierarchy of Needs," *Psychology Today* (May 23, 2012), https://www.psychologytoday.com/blog/hide-and-seek/201205/our-hierarchy-needs.

3. A. H. Maslow, "A Theory of Human Motivation," *Psychological Review*, 50 (1943): 370-396.

4. "Behaviors: How to Respond When Dementia Causes Unpredictable Behaviors," *The Alzheimer's Association*, rev. Jan.

17, page 4, https://www.alz.org/national/documents/brochure_behaviors.pdf.

5. Ibid., page 2.

Chapter 5

1. A. H. Maslow, "A Theory," 370-396.

2. Kassner and Jackson, "Determining Comparable."

3. M. P. Lawton and E. M. Brody, "Assessment of older people: Self-maintaining and instrumental activities of daily living." *Gerontologist,* 9 (1969) 179-186.

4. "Alzheimer's Stages: How the Disease Progresses," *Mayo Clinic,* 1998-2017, http://www.mayoclinic.org/alzheimers-stages/art-20048448?pg=2.

5. B. Reisberg, S. H. Ferris, M. J. de Leon, et. al., "The Global Deterioration Scale for Assessment of Primary Degenerative Dementia," *American Journal of Psychiatry* 139 (1982): 1136-1139.

6. Ann Louise Barrick, PhD, Joanne Rader, RN, MN, PMHNP, Beverly Hoeffer, DNSc, RN, et al., *Bathing without a Battle: Person-Directed Care of Individuals with Dementia* (New York: Springer Publishing Company, 2008).

7. "Alzheimer's Stages: How the Disease Progresses," *Mayo Clinic,* 1998-2017.

8. "Sleep Issues and Sundowning," The Alzheimer's Association, 2017, https://www.alz.org/care/alzheimers-dementia-sleep-issues-sundowning.asp.

9. "Does Medicare Cover Hospital Beds," Medicare.com, 2013, http://www.medicare.com/equipment-and-supplies/assistive-furniture/hospital-beds.html.

Chapter 6

1. A. H. Maslow, *Motivation and Personality* (New York: Harper & Row Publishers Inc., 1954), page 39.

2. Tom Slear, "The Deadliest Break: Hip fractures kill tens of thousands every year. Here's how to survive one," *AARP the Magazine* (October 2011), http://pubs.aarp.org/aarptm/201111?pg=30#.

3. "Early Signs of Dementia, Falls, Changes in Balance and Gait," The Alzheimer's Association, 2013, http://www.alzheimersreadingroom.com/2013/10/Dementia-Falling-Balance-Gait-Alzheimers.html.

4. "Staying Safe: Steps to Take for a Person with Dementia," The Alzheimer's Association, rev. Dec. 2016, http://www.alz.org/documents/national/brochure_stayingsafe.pdf.

5. U. S. Department of Health and Human Services, NIH National Institute on Aging, *Home Safety and Alzheimer's Disease*, July 25, 2017, https://www.nia.nih.gov/health/home-safety-and-alzheimers-disease.

6. "Medic Alert + Alzheimer's Association Safe Return," The Alzheimer's Association, 2017, http://www.alz.org/care/dementia-medic-alert-safe-return.asp.

7. "Comfort Zone," The Alzheimer's Association, 2017, http://www.alz.org/comfortzone/.

8. "About Project Lifesaver," *Project Lifesaver*, 2017 www.projectlifesaver.org.

9. State of Delaware, *Title II, Subchapter VII. Gold Alert Program for Certain Missing Persons,* 2008, http://delcode.delaware.gov/title11/c085/sc07/.

10. "Mild Cognitive Impairment," Alzheimer's Association website, https://www.alz.org/professionals_and_researchers_13518.asp.

11. Maslow, *Motivation,* pages 39-41.

12. "Long-Term Care Insurance: What You Should Know," *National Association of Insurance Commissioners (NAIC)*, 1990–2008, http://www.naic.org/documents/consumer_alert_ltc.htm.

13. Long-Term Care Insurance: The Risks and Benefits, by Joseph Matthews, Attorney, http://www.nolo.com/legal-encyclopedia/long-term-care-insurance-risks-benefits-30043.htm.

Chapter 7

1. Maslow, *Motivation,* pages 43-44.

2. "Changes to Your Relationship," Alzheimer's Association website, http://www.alz.org/care/alzheimers-dementia-relationship-changes.asp.

Chapter 8

1. Maslow, *Motivation,* page 45.

Chapter 9

1. Maslow, *Motivation,* page 46.

Chapter 10

1. Reisberg, et. al., "The Global Deterioration," 1136-1139.

2. "Current Alzheimer's Treatments," The Alzheimer's Association, 2017, https://www.alz.org/research/science/alzheimers_disease_treatments.asp.

3. "Stages and Behaviors," The Alzheimer's Association, 2017, https://www.alz.org/care/alzheimers-dementia-stages-behaviors.asp.

4. Joanne Koenig Coste, *Learning to Speak Alzheimer's: A Groundbreaking Approach for Everyone Dealing with the Disease* (New York: A Mariner Book, Houghton Mifflin, 2004), page 108.

5. Mary Ellen Geist, "The Healing Power of Music: For Alzheimer's Patients, Music Can Be Good Medicine," *AARP Bulletin/Real Possibilities* (July-August 2015).

6. Pfeiffer, "Treatment Options."

7. Puneet Narang, MD, et. al., "Antipsychotic Drugs: Sudden Cardiac Death among Elderly Patients," *Psychiatry (Edgmont)*, 10 (Oct 2010): 25-29, http://www.ncbi.nlm.nih.gov/pmc/articles/PMC2989835/.

Chapter 11

1. Ceridian Corporation, *Elder Care Handbook: Helping and Caring for Older Relatives,* 1999, page 22.

Chapter 12

1. Joseph Scriven, "What a Friend We Have in Jesus," public domain.

2. Dottie Rambo, "He Looked beyond My Fault (and Saw My Need), " John T. Benson Publishing Co., 1968.

3. Kirk Franklin, Fredrick Tackett, James Samuel Harris III, and Terry Lewis, "I Smile," 2011.

4. Luke 5:16, King James Bible.

5. Andrae Crouch, "Through It All," Manna Music Inc., 1999.

Chapter 13

1. The Alzheimer's Association, 2017, http.//www.alz.org.

2. "24/7 Helpline," The Alzheimer's Association, 2017, http://www.alz.org/we_can_help_24_7_helpline.asp.

3. "MedicAlert," The Alzheimer's Association.

4. "About TrialMatch, The Alzheimer's Association, 2017, https://www.alz.org/co/in_my_community_103098.asp.

5. National Institute on Aging, ADEAR, 2017, https://www.nia.nih.gov/alzheimers/about-adear-center.

6. The Alzheimer's Store, 2017, http://www.alzstore.com.

7. U. S. Department of Labor, Wage and Hour Division, *Fact Sheet #28: The Family and Medical Leave Act*, 2012, *http://www.dol.gov/whd/regs/compliance/whdfs28.pdf.*

Chapter 14

1. "Communication: Tips for Successful Communication during All Stages of Alzheimer's Disease," The Alzheimer's Association, May 2017, http://www.alz.org/national/documents/brochure_communication.pdf.

2. Coste, *Learning to Speak.*

Chapter 16

1. "Legal Plans: Assisting a Person with Dementia in Planning for the Future," rev. Feb. 17, The Alzheimer's Association, http://www.alz.org/national/documents/brochure_legalplans.pdf.

Chapter 17

1. "Compare Long-Term Care Costs across the United States," *Genworth*, 2017, https://www.genworth.com/corporate/about-genworth/industry-expertise/cost-of-care.html.

2. Ibid.

3. U. S. Department of Health and Human Services, *Other State Programs*, 2017, https://longtermcare.acl.gov/medicare-medicaid-more/state-based-programs.html.

4. U. S. Centers for Medicare & Medicaid Services, *Your Medicare Coverage, Skilled Nursing Facility (SNF) Care*, 2017, https://www.medicare.gov/coverage/skilled-nursing-facility-care.html.

5. U. S. Department of Health and Human Services, *State Medicaid Programs,* 2017, https://longtermcare.acl.gov/medicare-medicaid-more/medicaid/index.html.

6. U. S. Centers for Medicare & Medicaid Services, *How Can I Pay for Nursing Home Care?* 2017, https://www.medicare.gov/what-medicare-covers/part-a/paying-for-nursing-home-care.html.

7. *2017 Alzheimer's Disease Facts,* The Alzheimer's Association, page 51.

8. Agency for Healthcare Research and Quality, U. S. Department of Health & Human Services, *Comparison of Characteristics of Nursing Homes and Other Residential Long-Term Care Settings for People with Dementia,* November 2, 2011, https://effectivehealthcare.ahrq.gov/topics/dementia-nursing-home-characteristics/research-protocol/.

9. CDC Vital and Health Statistics, *Long-Term Care Services in the United States: 2013,* Dec. 2013, http://www.cdc.gov/nchs/data/nsltcp/long_term_care_services_2013.pdf.

10. Agency for Healthcare, *Comparison of Characteristics.*

11. CDC Vital, *Long-Term Care.*

12. Ibid.

13. "NHPCO's Facts and Figures: Hospice Care in America," National Hospice and Palliative Care Organization, 2015, http://www.nhpco.org/hospice-statistics-research-press-room/facts-hospice-and-palliative-care.

14. "Compare Long Term," *Genworth.*

15. "Alzheimer's and Dementia Care Costs: Facts & Figures," Senior Homes.com, 2017, http://www.seniorhomes.com/p/alzheimers-care-costs/.

16. "What Is Alzheimer's Memory Care?" A Place for Mom, 2017, http://www.aplaceformom.com/alzheimers-care#services.

17. "Compare Long Term," *Genworth.*

18. "Hospice and End-of-Life Options and Costs," Debt.org, 2017 https://www.debt.org/medical/hospice-costs/.

19. NIH, National Institute on Aging, *Long-Term Care: Paying for Care*, 2017, https://www.nia.nih.gov/health/paying-care.

20. "Hospice Care," National Hospice and Palliative Care Organization, 04/03/2017, https://www.nhpco.org/about/hospice-care.

21. "Residential Care," The Alzheimer's Association, 2017, http://www.alz.org/care/alzheimers-dementia-residential-facilities.asp#checklist.

22. U. S. Centers for Medicare & Medicaid Services, *Find a Nursing Home*, 2017,

23. https://www.medicare.gov/nursinghomecompare/search.html. "Nursing Homes Ratings," *U.S. News and World Report*, 2017, http://health.usnews.com/best-nursing-homes.

Chapter 18

1. *2017 Alzheimer's Disease Facts*, The Alzheimer's Association, page 51.

2. Personal Care: Assisting a Person with Middle- or Late-Stage Dementia with Daily Needs," The Alzheimer's Association, rev. Dec. 16, http://www.alz.org/national/documents/brochure_personalcare.pdf.

3. Nancy L. Mace and Peter V. Rabins, *The 36-Hour Day: A Family Guide to Caring for People Who Have Alzheimer Disease, Related Dementias, and Memory Loss* (Baltimore: Johns Hopkins University Press, 2017).

4. "essentiALZ", The Alzheimer's Association, 2017, http://www.alz.org/essentialz/.

5. Department of Health and Human Services, Adult Day Care, Eldercare Locator, 2015, http://www.eldercare.gov/Eldercare. NET/Public/Resources/Factsheets/Adult_Day_Care.aspx.

6. Department of Health and Human Services, Home Health Care, 2/6/2017, http://www.eldercare.gov/eldercare.net/public/ resources/factsheets/home_health_care.aspx.

7. Ibid.

8. 24/7 Helpline, The Alzheimer's Association, 2017, http://www. alz.org/we_can_help_24_7_helpline.asp.

Chapter 19

1. "Mild Cognitive Impairment," Alzheimer's Association website.

Chapter 20

1. Wesley Patrick, "Assisted Living Facilities," Caregiver.com, http://www.caregiver.com/articles/general/assisted_living_ facilities.htm.

2. Ibid.

Chapter 21

1. Daniel L. Paris, MSW, "Alzheimer's Disease Special Care Units," Caregiver.com, http://www.caregiver.com/channels/alz/articles/ alz_special_care_unit.htm.

Chapter 22

1. Wesley Patrick, "Nursing Home Care," Caregiver.com, http:// www.caregiver.com/channels/ltc/articles/nursing_home_care. htm.

2. U. S. Centers for Medicare & Medicaid Services, *Nursing Home Toolkit: Nursing Homes—A Guide for Medicaid Beneficiaries' Families and Helpers,* November 2015, page 6. https://www.

cms.gov/Medicare-Medicaid-Coordination/Fraud-Prevention/
Medicaid-Integrity-Education/Downloads/nursinghome-
beneficiary-booklet.pdf.

Chapter 23

1. "Medicare Hospice Benefits," Hospicenet.org, http://hospicenet.
   org/html/medicare.html.
2. U. S. Centers for Medicare & Medicaid Services, *Medicare Hospice Benefits*, April 2017 https://www.medicare.gov/Pubs/
   pdf/02154-Medicare-Hospice-Benefits.PDF.

Chapter 25

1. Win Thompkins, "The Leaning Tree," Uncle Win's Music Productions, Inc., 2009.
2. "10 Symptoms of Caregiver Stress," The Alzheimer's Association, 2017, http://www.alz.org/care/alzheimers-dementia-caregiver-stress-burnout.asp.
3. *2017 Alzheimer's Disease Facts*, The Alzheimer's Association, page 40.
4. *2009 Alzheimer's Disease Facts and Figures,* The Alzheimer's Association, 2009, page 38, *https://www.alz.org/national/documents/report_alzfactsfigures2009.pdf.*
5. *2014 Alzheimer's Disease Facts and Figures,* The Alzheimer's Association, page 34, *https://www.alz.org/downloads/facts_figures_2014.pdf.*
6. *2017 Alzheimer's Disease Facts*, The Alzheimer's Association, page 11.
7. *2017 Alzheimer's Disease Facts*, The Alzheimer's Association, page 12.
8. Osorio, et al., "Sleep-disordered Breathing."

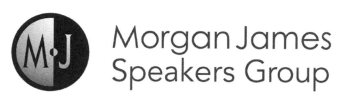

Morgan James
Speakers Group

www.TheMorganJamesSpeakersGroup.com

We connect Morgan James published
authors with live and online events
and audiences who will benefit
from their expertise.

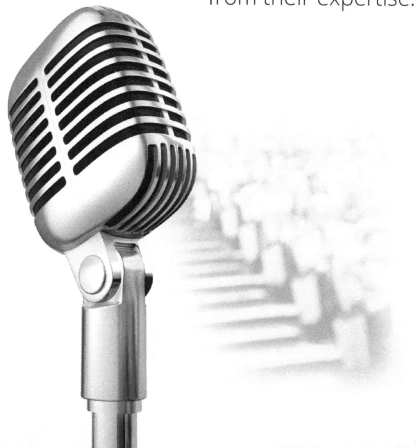